Patient Safety and Hospital Accreditation

Sharon Myers, RN, MSN, MSB, FACHE, CPHQ, CHCQM, CPHRM, graduated from Johns Hopkins University School of Nursing, with both a master of science in nursing health systems management and a master of science in business.

She is currently the quality management officer for the VA MidSouth Healthcare Network (VISN 9) in Nashville where she provides oversight to six health care facilities, ensuring utilization management, continuous survey readiness, systems redesign, and data-management activities, support high-quality patient care and is an adjunct associate nursing professor at Vanderbilt University School of Nursing.

Prior to her VA career, Myers worked as the director of quality management at the King Abdulaziz Medical City in Saudi Arabia and successfully led that facility through its first Joint Commission accreditation. She also served as senior consultant to the Makkah Region Quality Program and the Central Board of Accreditation of Healthcare Institutions in Saudi Arabia, where she assisted in the development of the first *Hospital Standards Manual* which was approved by the Ministry of Health for implementation. Subsequently, she assisted Central Board of Accreditation for Healthcare Institutions (CBAHI) in developing their national survey process. She was the assistant director of nursing at Johns Hopkins Bayview Care Center in Baltimore, where she led nursing groups to develop a career ladder for nursing assistants in long-term care which won an "innovations in nursing practice" award. In addition to the quality-improvement positions she held in Saudi Arabia, she has also been a nursing education coordinator, clinical educator, and nursing supervisor. She has owned an independent consulting firm which developed curriculum for cross-training medical–surgical nurses for critical care and developed self-learning modules approved by the Florida State Board. She served as a Captain in the U.S. Air Force, serving three tours of duty, one of which was overseas.

She is a recognized international speaker on indicators and measurement, quality concepts, and patient safety. In addition, she has been a guest lecturer at Johns Hopkins School of Nursing and at King Abdulaziz University in Saudi Arabia.

She holds numerous national certifications and memberships in health care management, quality management, and risk management. She has authored many instructional articles, and is a published author in the fields of accreditation and patient safety.

When not on travel, Myers resides outside of Nashville, Tennessee, with her husband, John.

Patient Safety and Hospital Accreditation

A Model for Ensuring Success

Sharon Ann Myers, RN, MSN, MSB, FACHE,
CPHQ, CHCQM, CPHRM

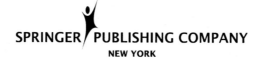

SPRINGER PUBLISHING COMPANY
NEW YORK

Springer Publishing Company, LLC
11 West 42nd Street
New York, NY 10036
www.springerpub.com

Acquisitions Editor: Allan Graubard
Production Editor: Michael Lisk
Composition: S4Carlisle Publishing Services

ISBN: 978-0-8261-0639-1
E-book ISBN: 978-0-8261-0640-7

11 12 13/ 5 4 3 2 1

The author and the publisher of this Work have made every effort to use sources believed to be reliable to provide information that is accurate and compatible with the standards generally accepted at the time of publication. The author and publisher shall not be liable for any special, consequential, or exemplary damages resulting, in whole or in part, from the readers' use of, or reliance on, the information contained in this book. The publisher has no responsibility for the persistence or accuracy of URLs for external or third-party Internet Web sites referred to in this publication and does not guarantee that any content on such Web sites is, or will remain, accurate or appropriate.

Library of Congress Cataloging-in-Publication Data
Myers, Sharon.
  Patient safety and hospital accreditation : a model for ensuring success / Sharon Ann Myers.
      p. ; cm.
  Includes bibliographical references.
  ISBN 978-0-8261-0639-1
  ISBN 978-0-8261-0640-7 (e-book)
I. Title.
  [DNLM: 1. Safety Management—standards. 2. Accreditation—standards.
3. Hospitals—standards. 4. Models, Nursing. 5. Patient Care—standards. WX 185]
  LC classification not assigned
  362.11028'9—dc23
                                    2011038875

Printed in the United States of America by Gasch Printing

This book is dedicated to my husband, John, who has supported my professional and personal goals for the past 30 years. He has encouraged me to think outside of the conventional boxes, to not accept what is, but to strive for "what should be" to make health care trustworthy for our patients and staff.

Contents

Preface

First do no harm. It has been more than 10 years since the Institute of Medicine's report *To Err is Human: Building a Safer Health System* was published and patient safety became a priority in the United States and internationally.

The goal of this book is to provide a model for consideration when leading patient safety and accreditation initiatives. The *Myers Model for Patient Safety and Accreditation* is the first time that current evidence has been presented within a model that assists strategic planning to sustain or to gain accreditation with high levels of patient safety.

There are five sections in this book. Section I covers the key concepts related to hospital accreditation and patient safety, important milestones of each, then branches out into the global view. Interviews with three major leaders of health care accreditation programs are included: Joint Commission, Accreditation Canada, and the Australian Council on Healthcare Standards (ACHS). Each leader shared their views on key aspects of patient safety in relation to their own accreditation program. Joint Commission's leader, Dr. Paul Schyve, senior vice president, discussed the Hand Hygiene Project at the *Center for Transforming Healthcare* (subsidiary of the Joint Commission). He also spoke about how the Patient Safety Advisory Group is tackling issues such as worker fatigue. Wendy Nicklin, president and CEO of Accreditation Canada, discussed standards that measure the Quality of WorkLife. Accreditation Canada administers a *Worklife Pulse Survey* every 3 years as part of the accreditation process. In Canada, a positive worklife culture is considered a strategic priority. Brian W. Johnston, chief executive of the ACHS, discussed how they use an internationally recognized Evaluation and Quality Improvement Program (EQuIP) that encourages progressively higher standards of performance through a 4-year EQuIP cycle. ACHS has a number of indicator sets that are specialty specific that measure adverse events.

Section II sets up the foundation of why a model is needed when implementing patient safety and accreditation programs. This section covers some of the current challenges in health care with emphasis on concepts of reliability that are related to patient safety. Outdated organizational architecture is discussed along with various structures that may enhance work at the unit (microsystem) level. Finally, a general overview of the *Myers Model for Patient Safety and Accreditation* is presented. The model presents a systems approach that should be used when initiating patient safety and/or accreditation initiatives. Every element within the model is interrelated with the other components. The three levels of organizational architecture are presented: design at the leadership level (system), the unit level (microsystem), and the individual level. All three levels must be aligned with the other elements within the model to achieve the aims of the system.

Section III presents the three levels in detail with current evidence for each level. There is great emphasis placed on design at the leadership level. If the leadership is dysfunctional, it will negatively affect all of the other elements in the model and make it difficult, if not impossible, to achieve the aims of the system. Design at the unit (microsystem) level is aligned with the other elements within the model, and current research is presented for evaluation when developing and maintaining effective outcomes. Design at the individual level is aligned with all the other elements within the model, including nursing leadership, making it clear how the *Myers Model for Patient Safety and Accreditation* assists in creating and sustaining an enriched environment of professional practice that ensures engagement of nursing staff.

Section IV provides an overview of reporting systems within the United States and covers two essential tools that are used to ensure patient safety: root-cause analysis and failure mode and effects analysis.

The last section contains recommendations for consideration to accrediting bodies and to health care organizations, which may enhance their patient safety and accreditation efforts. This section summarizes previous material presented and reinforces the new aims statement. *ZERO is the number and NOW is the time.* "No preventable harm to patients or staff" is the goal for high–reliability health care organizations and the time to start working toward that goal is *NOW*.

I

Overview of Hospital Accreditation and Patient Safety

1

Introduction to Concepts of Hospital Accreditation and Patient Safety

OVERVIEW

When patients are admitted to the hospital, they put their trust in health care professionals to do the right thing, on time, all of the time. Health care systems that are accredited demonstrate to the public that they have maintained compliance with a set of standards that provides the public at least some reassurance that quality and patient safety standards are being met. Unfortunately, even in accredited health care organizations, patients are harmed by medical errors every day.

Accreditation is increasingly being utilized as a key driver for implementation of patient safety efforts to reduce patient harm caused by medical errors.

There are many definitions of accreditation; however, there is a general consensus on the following key concepts:

- Accreditation is usually a voluntary process.
- Accreditation's evaluation process is external.
- Accreditation involves the use of dynamic standards organized into three domains.
- Accreditation's standards have the potential to achieve optimum performance.

Accreditation Is Usually a Voluntary Process

Accreditation for health care organizations is seen as a voluntary or legal requirement in many countries. In the United States, accreditation programs are voluntary and must be approved by the Centers for Medicare and Medicaid Services (CMS) programs for the health care organization to participate in and receive payment from the Medicare or Medicaid program. CMS may grant the accrediting organization "deeming" authority, in which case, the health care organization would not be subject to Medicare's routine survey and certification process.

Accreditation's Evaluation Process Is External

The fact that the evaluation process is external to the organization ensures greater objectivity than if the evaluation were internal.

Having outsiders with no relationship to the health care organization assess the level of performance according to an agreed-on set of standards is critical for accreditation.

The surveyors are health care professionals carefully selected for their subject matter expertise. This becomes a form of external peer review when the surveyors are matched to clinical and nonclinical areas according to their expertise.

The Accreditation Process Involves Standards

Standards are developed through a consensus process and peer review. Professional organizations, various stakeholder groups, and expert panels are all used in writing standards in which the expected performance is measured in the accreditation process by survey methods.

Standards Are Dynamic and Are Organized Into Three Domains

Standards are not static. They are continually revised as new knowledge emerges. Health care standards are organized into the three domains of structure, process, and outcome based on Donabedian's model (Donabedian, 1988).

Increasingly, patient safety standards are being integrated into the Joint Commission accreditation requirements. According to the Joint Commission (2010), almost 50 percent of their standards are directly related to patient safety.

FIGURE 1.1
Hospital accreditation potential level of quality through application
of continuous quality improvement (CQI).

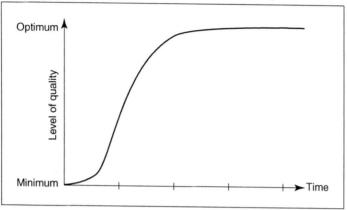

OPTIMAL ACHIEVEMENT OF STANDARDS

Accreditation organizations encourage health care organizations to achieve optimal standards through the application of continuous quality improvement (CQI) concepts. Through the application of CQI concepts, an organization is able to progress from its existing level of performance to the optimal level of standards compliance (see Figure 1.1).

Ten years ago, optimal level of achievement looked very different than it does today. For example, accepted thresholds for hospital-acquired infections for central line–associated bloodstream infections were set before any improvement project was initiated. There was a general complacency and acceptance that many adverse events were related to complications beyond the provider's control.

Expectations are different now. For example, there is the implementation across the United States of the Institute for Healthcare Improvement's (IHI's) 5 Million Lives Campaign. Here, through consistent implementation of the central line bundles, central line–related infections have been dramatically reduced to zero.

PATIENT SAFETY DEFINED

Errors that result in patient injury are sometimes called preventable adverse events, which means that the injury resulted from a medical intervention and not the patient's underlying disease state. An example of a preventable adverse event is if a patient were to receive 10 times the normal dose of an anticoagulant resulting in death.

The Agency for Healthcare Research and Quality (AHRQ) describes patient safety as "freedom from accidental or preventable injuries produced by medical care" (AHRQ, n.d.-a). Health care organizations are expected to provide safe care and do no harm. Luckily, all medical errors do not result in preventable adverse events, either through chance or timely intervention.

An example of a medical error in which no harm occurred because of chance is when the patient receives the wrong diagnostic test because of misidentification; however, no harm occurred because the diagnostic test (by chance) was noninvasive with minimal risk.

An example of no harm occurring because of timely intervention is when a nurse administers double the dosage of a narcotic, which depresses respirations of a patient; however, she recognizes her error and the patient receives timely intervention through administration of Narcan, which reverses the narcotic effects quickly.

COMMON THEMES OF PATIENT SAFETY

Patient safety concepts involve culture, communication, high-reliability organizations (HROs), systems thinking, human factors, reliability, evidence-based medicine, reporting systems, and use of tools such as failure modes, effects analysis, and root cause analysis (RCA). All of these concepts reside under the umbrella of CQI and continuous and consistent leadership.

Culture

Improving the culture of safety is an essential component of preventing or reducing errors as well as improving overall health care quality.

Unfortunately, even though culture is an essential component for patient safety, the AHRQ has reported wide variation in patient safety cultures in hospitals across the United States.

According to the IHI (n.d.-a), "In a culture of safety, people are not merely encouraged to work toward change; they take action when it is needed."

The AHRQ (n.d.-b) states that the culture of patient safety comprises the following key features:

- There is acknowledgment of the high-risk nature of an organiza-tion's activities and the determination to achieve consistently safe operations.

  Health care organizations now acknowledge that providing care to patients is risky and are increasingly becoming determined to achieve higher degrees of safety.
- There is a blame-free environment and individuals are able to report errors or near misses without fear of reprimand or punishment.

  The term *blame-free* was misunderstood initially to mean that no person would be accountable for his or her actions. The term used now is just *culture* (as in a "culture of justice"), where reckless be-havior is not tolerated; however, no one is punished for making an honest mistake.
- There is encouragement for collaboration across ranks and disci-plines to seek solutions to patient safety problems.
- In hospitals, collaboration is challenging because of conflicting cultures, politics, and organizational architectures.
- The organization commits resources to address safety concerns. Hospitals have shrinking budgets and numerous competing de-mands for money expenditures, which is especially challenging when expensive capital expenditures are required.

There is an increasing interest in measuring patient safety culture within health care organizations, and accrediting bodies such as Joint Commission are including patient safety culture as a requirement for measurement and improvement.

Communication

Communication deficiencies in large complex systems are one of the primary contributing causes for medical errors.

The Controlled Risk Insurance Company of Vermont (CRICO/ RMF), the patient and medical malpractice company that has served the Harvard medical community since 1976, states that medical errors can occur when individuals from different backgrounds or health care disciplines have different communication styles that the organization does not accommodate.

CRICO further states that role conflict or confusion occurs when any member of a health care team is uncertain about the specific role he or she is expected to fill, or when he or she is confused about the role and responsibilities of other team members. Role confusion results in communication problems, which can lead to medical errors.

There are many communication interventions for health care systems that assist in building a safer environment for patient care (CRICO/RMF, n.d.).

Some examples include Crew Resource Management (CRM), which was adopted from the aviation industry in 1979. The concept was used in the aviation industry to address the role that human errors played in airplane crashes to achieve flights that were safe and effective.

CRM involves team training on the limitations of human performance. Staff are taught about cognitive errors and the influence that stressors such as fatigue, work overload, and emergent situations can have on the frequency of errors. Staff are taught to speak up using inquiry and advocacy methods and communication techniques, including conflict resolution (Pizza, Goldfarb, & Nash, 2001).

IHI (n.d.-b) presented the Situation-Background, Assessment-Recommendation (SBAR) as another technique for communication between members of the health care team. This involves a standardized method to communicate a patient's condition during handovers and is available at http://www.ihi.org/knowledge/Pages/Tools/SBARToolkit.aspx.

Team training involves effective communication and team functioning skills, which must be learned in order for the staff to gain competencies. Team training is described as "the application of instructional strategies based on well-tested tools (e.g., simulators, lectures, and videos) to a specific set of competencies" (AHRQ, n.d.-c).

High-Reliability Organizations (HROs)

> HROs are organizations with systems in place that are exceptionally consistent in accomplishing their goals and avoiding potentially catastrophic errors. (AHRQ, 2008)

The industries first to embrace HRO concepts were those in which past failures led to catastrophic consequences: airplane crashes, nuclear reactor meltdowns, and other such disasters.

These industries discovered it was essential to identify weak danger signals and to respond to these signals strongly so that system functioning could be maintained and disasters could be avoided.

Basic characteristics for HROs applied to hospitals include the following basic concepts:

Hypercomplexity—Hospitals are extremely complex systems in which multiple sequential and nonsequential tasks are carried out by multiple staff to produce outcomes. As any health care worker will tell you, "There is no such thing as a simple operation."

All operations depend on numerous staff to perform their roles perfectly and at the right time to produce effective outcomes. An error by just one team member can easily cascade into disastrous outcomes.

Tight coupling–Interdependent tasks—These are tasks performed rapidly that require perfect coordination to deliver the right care to the right patient at the right time. Operating rooms and critical care areas have tight coupling.

Extreme hierarchical differentiation—During times of crisis, authority is granted to the person with the best skill set to do the job. An example of this would be two staff members, a nurse and a physician, responding to a cardiac arrest; the nurse is ACLS certified and the physician is not: the nurse leads the code.

Multiple decision makers in a complex communication network—Within a hospital setting, many people make decisions regarding the patient's care. *Coordination and effective communication* between all decision makers is essential.

High degree of accountability—HROs have a high degree of accountability when errors occur with severe consequences. Hospitals do not routinely deal in mass injuries such as those resulting from a plane crash; however, the medical profession and legal system hold medical professionals to a higher accountability standard when adverse events occur.

Need for immediate and frequent feedback—Continuous feedback is essential because it enables the team to make rapid adjustments when unpredictable events occur. Also, it assists the team to discern what is important to act on versus what is not as important and can be handled later. When staff is afraid to voice their concerns for patient safety, the patient is subjected to serious risk.

The final HRO characteristic relates to *compressed time constraints*— The patient requires care 24 hours a day/7 days a week. When resources are stretched (such as when there is a shortage of nurses), important tasks may be delegated to ancillary staff during a shift or carried over for the next shift's nurse to carry out. Accurate communication of the patient's needs is necessary to prevent adverse events.

Systems Thinking

It takes a community of diverse medical staff, each performing his or her piece of a complex process perfectly, to provide safe patient care. This is not an easy thing to do and requires systems thinking to integrate the pieces of care into a holistic framework in which to target patient-safety efforts.

Hospitals are complex systems. Health care systems are composed of multiple, interrelated activities called processes that result in patient outcomes on a daily basis. When human error occurs, a chain of subsequent events similar to a domino effect can result in patient harm.

An example of a domino effect is when a patient arrives in the emergency room and the physician experiences a delay in obtaining the patient's prior medical record. The physician then makes an error in prescribing a treatment because he or she did not have the needed information about the patient's past medical history to make a sound clinical decision.

Another example is when there is a shortage of made-up beds in the intensive care unit because of reduced housekeeping staff. Now, there are delays in admissions to the intensive care unit due to the delays in housekeeping staff cleaning the beds. This shortage of housekeeping staff created a domino effect which has the potential to cause an adverse event.

Simple solutions are not effective for complex problem solving when there are multiple, interrelated activities that result in a range of potential outcomes for patients. Senge (1990) described systems thinking as "a conceptual framework, as a body of knowledge and tools that has been developed over the past fifty years, to make the full patterns clearer and to help us see how to change them effectively."

Senge identified systems thinking as one of the essentials an organization must have to build a learning organization, along with personal mastery, mental models, building a shared vision, and team learning.

He argued that one of the key problems in management is that simplistic frameworks are applied to complex systems, which results in a focus on only the parts rather than the whole, and produces less than optimal results.

The other difficulty lies in the time line related to cause and effect. In complex systems, many times it takes years for the full effects of multiple, interrelated activities to fully play out.

When a nurse makes a medication error, the easy and simple solution is to counsel the nurse and reinforce the policy of checking two patient identifiers. However, this solution is not effective because nothing in the system design changed to prevent the occurrence from happening again.

The Institute of Medicine (IOM, 2001) stated that complex adaptive systems have both the freedom and the capacity to respond to stimuli in many different and fundamentally unpredictable ways resulting in either innovation or error. The IOM provides the following six aims for health care systems:

- Safe: Patients should not be harmed by the care that is intended to help them.
- Effective: Care should be based on scientific knowledge and offered to all who could benefit and not to those not likely to benefit.
- Patient centered: Care should be respectful of and responsive to individual patient preferences, needs, and values.
- Timely: Waits and sometimes harmful delays in care should be reduced both for those who receive care and for those who give care.
- Efficient: Care should be given without wasting equipment, supplies, ideas, and energy.
- Equitable: Care should not vary in quality because of personal characteristics such as gender, ethnicity, geographic location, and socioeconomic status.

Achieving a higher level of quality is essential as a first step in improving the quality of care overall; this requires new designs of systems that prevent error and minimize harm.

Human Factors

The field of human factors is used to analyze the environment and interfaces between the human operator and the system to produce safer systems of care.

Licht, Polzella, and Boff (n.d.) researched the broadening of the term *human factor* and noted that there appears to be a broadening of the focus with application to many fields. The authors stated that originally the focus of human factors was

> On the design of military man-machine systems. It is obvious that this focus has expanded to include private industry and consumer products as well. Thus the field has moved from a discipline born in a postwar militarily orientated engineering environment to a more global manufacturing and consumer oriented environment. (n.d.)

Kohn, Corrigan, and Donaldson (2000) acknowledged that human factors are just beginning to be applied within health care.

Reliability

The IHI (n.d.-c) defines reliability theory as "a scientific method of evaluating, calculating, and improving the overall reliability of a complex system." These concepts have been embraced by and used effectively in industries such as manufacturing, nuclear power, and aircraft carriers. Using reliability concepts, these industries have improved the rate at which they consistently produce appropriate outcomes and prevent adverse events.

Reliability theory, when applied to health care, has the potential to help reduce defects in care or care processes and increase the consistency with which appropriate care is delivered and thus to improve patient outcomes.

Unfortunately, health care is not reliable yet. Indeed, the health care provided to patients has a long way to go to reach the level of success attained by HROs. Remember: If an audit of care provided shows 90 percent compliance with standards, this means that 1 out of every 10 patients did not receive the optimum care that the system designed. One patient out of 10 may suffer an adverse event because of the low reliability of the process designed by the system.

Evidence-Based Medicine

Sackett and Rosenberg (1995) explained evidence-based medicine (EBM) as the ability to track down, critically appraise and incorporate evidence into clinical practice. They feel that as studies of valid evidence increase, so does the requirement for the medical community to develop the skills necessary to understand, evaluate, and make best use of that evidence for patients.

One of the benefits of EBM is that greater consistency of treatment appropriate to the patient's symptoms might be achieved. There is wide variation in the treatment provided by physicians to patients (Wennberg & Gittelsohn, 1982), and variation is a source of medical errors that can lead to adverse events. Recently, the AHRQ stated that

> Every day, millions of Americans receive high-quality health care that helps to maintain or restore their health and ability to function. However, far too many do not. Quality problems

are reflected in a wide variation in the use of health care services, underuse of some services, overuse of other services, and misuse of services, including an unacceptable level of errors. (n.d.-d)

The goal of patient safety applied to EBM is to deliver the right treatment at the right time, to the right patient, all of the time. If the patient receives the right care only 90 percent of the time, that is simply not enough to be an acceptable standard of care.

Reporting Systems

The medical community, mortality and morbidity conferences, grand rounds, and peer review all currently share the same shortcomings: a lack of human factors and thinking about systems.

This leads to these review processes having a narrow focus on individual performance to the exclusion of contributory team and larger social issues. This lack of a systems focus also leads to hindsight bias, which is the tendency to search for errors rather than for the numerous causes of error induction (Barach, 2000).

Reporting systems have the potential to provide information that can be used to prevent future adverse events from occurring and also to enhance learning of staff; however, voluntary reporting systems have their own set of problems.

Despite aviation's success stories, physicians remain reluctant to use reporting systems. The studies have demonstrated that physicians are reluctant to participate in programs to report medical errors and that underreporting of adverse events may be as high as 96 percent (Harper & Helmreich, 2005).

The AHRQ's findings suggest that the success of a reporting system is determined by the attitudes and perceptions of frontline care providers. Prior to implementing an event-reporting system, there needs to be an assessment of the opinions of care providers to identify critical barriers to reporting. Those issues should be dealt with prior to implementing a reporting system.

Use of Tools

Proper tools are a necessity. Abraham Maslow (2009) once said, "If the only tool you have is a hammer, you will see every problem as a nail."

The world does not operate in a linear fashion. When managers continue to solve complex problems with linear action plans, the results are often not as intended. What is needed is a radically new tool kit.

This new tool kit would contain new skills. The new skills would be congruent with the "new paradigm view" of organizations as unpredictable, interactive, living systems, rather than being viewed as machine-like systems.

There are numerous approaches to using tools for every aspect of patient safety, from the basic tools of how to perform a credible RCA of an adverse event to how to perform a health care failure modes and effects analysis.

Checklists are increasingly being used in health care as one of the tools to help ensure patient safety. An example of this is the central line checklist, a tool whose use has resulted in a dramatic reduction in the prevention of central line infections (Pronovost et al., 2006).

There is also the World Alliance Surgical Safety Checklist (World Alliance for Patient Safety, 2008), which was developed to assist in minimizing the most common and avoidable risks for surgical patients.

In this light, there are free starter kits such as Botwinick, Bisognano, and Haraden's *Leadership Guide to Patient Safety* (2006) that the IHI offers online. In fact, there are numerous online resources for tools to use when implementing a patient safety program, such as those listed in Table 1.1.

TABLE 1.1
Online Tools for Patient Safety

WEBSITE	WHAT'S IN IT
www.ahrq.gov/qual/pips/ www.ahrq.gov/qual/pstools.htm www.ahrq.gov/qual/errorsix.htm www.ahrq.gov/qual/hospsurvey09/ teamstepps.ahrq.gov/ abouttoolsmaterials.htm	Agency for Healthcare Research and Quality (AHRQ) Domains for tools; extensive Hotlinks available: setting and user, patient safety issue area/user and patient safety goals. Also contains team training tools and patient safety culture survey information
www.mgma.com/pppsahome/	Medical Group Management Association (MGMA) Tools for assisting physicians to assess their practice
www.patientsafety.gov/ safetytopics.html	United States Department of Veterans Affairs Resources for how to conduct RCA/FMEA and numerous tools to implement programs such as falls prevention, hand hygiene, and so on

TABLE 1.1 (*Continued*)

WEBSITE	WHAT'S IN IT
www.ihi.org/IHI/Topics/PatientSafety/SafetyGeneral/Tools/	Institute for Health Care Improvement (IHI) Leadership tools, communication HFMEA, trigger tools, general tools, and so on
www.healthpartners.com/files/34649.pdf	Health Partners: Ambulatory Care Ambulatory care tool kit
www.ismp.org/tools/abbreviations/	Institute for Safe Medicine Practices (ISMP) Medication safety tools: error-prone abbreviation list
www.nursingleadershipcongress.com/ToolKit.asp	Nursing Congress Leadership tools for implementing patient safety; includes financial aspects of patient safety
www.ccforpatientsafety.org/patient-safety-solutions/	Joint Commission in collaboration with WHO Nine patient safety solutions
www.psnet.ahrq.gov/browseResourceType.aspx?resourceTypeID=203	Patient safety network: AHRQ 134 resources and tools for patient safety
www.rmf.harvard.edu/patient-safety-strategies/communication-teamwork/articles/teamwork-as-a-tool.aspx	Controlled Risk Insurance Company/Risk Management Foundation Team training tools
teamstepps.ahrq.gov/	AHRQ Evidence-based team training tools
www.dana-farber.org/pat/patient-safety/patient-safety-resources/patient-rounding-toolkit.html	Dana Farber Patient rounding tool kit, patient safety resources
www.npsf.org/paf/pafrg/	National Patient Safety Foundation (NPSF) Resources for patient safety
www.who.int/patientsafety/safesurgery/en/	Patient safety surgical checklist and other resources
www.who.int/patientsafety/education/curriculum/download/en/index.html	World Health Organization International (WHO) Curriculum for patient safety for WHO International medical students
www.massmed.org/AM/Template.cfm?Section=Home6&TEMPLATE=/CM/HTMLDisplay.cfm&CONTENTID=3925	Massachusetts Medical Society (MassMed) Patient safety curriculum

CONCLUSION

Accreditation programs are usually voluntary in nature and involve external peer review. Standards are the foundation for accreditation programs and they evolve over time, becoming increasingly challenging as compliance to the established set of standards is obtained. Standards have the potential to generate optimal performance.

Patient safety concepts involve culture, communication, systems thinking, human factors, reliability, EBM, reporting systems, and the use of tools. Increasingly, patient safety concepts are being included in accreditation standards.

REFERENCES

Agency for Healthcare Research and Quality. (2008). *Becoming a high reliability organization: Operational advice for hospital leaders.* Retrieved from http://www.ahrq.gov/qual/hroadvice/

Agency for Healthcare Research and Quality. (n.d.-a). *Agency for healthcare research and quality: Glossary.* Retrieved from http://psnet.ahrq.gov/glossary.aspx

Agency for Healthcare Research and Quality. (n.d.-b). *Improving health care quality: Fact sheet.* Retrieved from http://www.ahrq.gov/news/qualfact.htm

Agency for Healthcare Research and Quality. (n.d.-c). *Medical teamwork and patient safety.* Retrieved from http://www.ahrq.gov/qual/medteam/med team2.htm#training

Agency for Healthcare Research and Quality Patient Safety Network. (n.d.-d). *Safety culture.* Retrieved from http://www.psnet.ahrq.gov/primer.aspx?primerID=5

Barach, P. (2000). Reporting and preventing medical mishaps: Lessons from nonmedical near miss reporting systems. *British Medical Journal, 320,* P759–P763.

Botwinick, L., Bisognano, M., & Haraden, C. (2006). *Leadership guide to patient safety.* Retrieved from http://www.ihi.org/IHI/Results/WhitePapers/LeadershipGuidetoPatientSafetyWhitePaper.htm

CRICO/RMF. (n.d.). *Teamwork as a tool for patient safety.* Retrieved from http://www.rmf.harvard.edu/patient-safety-strategies/communication-teamwork/articles/teamwork-as-a-tool.aspx

Donabedian, A. (1988). The quality of care: How can it be assessed? *Journal of the American Medical Association, 260,* 1743–1748.

Harper, M. L., & Helmreich, R. L. (2005). *Identifying barriers to the success of a reporting system.* Retrieved from http://www.ncbi.nlm.nih.gov/books/NBK20544/

Institute for Healthcare Improvement. (n.d.-a). *Develop a culture of safety.* Retrieved from http://www.ihi.org/knowledge/Pages/Changes/DevelopaCultureofSafety.aspx

Institute for Healthcare Improvement. (n.d.-b) *SBAR technique for communication: A situational briefing model.* Retrieved from http://www.ihi.org/IHI/Topics/PatientSafety/SafetyGeneral/Tools/SBARTechniquefor CommunicationASituationalBriefingModel.htm

Institute for Healthcare Improvement. (n.d.-c) *Reliability.* Retrieved from http://www.ihi.org/IHI/Topics/Reliability/

Institute of Medicine. (2001). *Crossing the quality chasm: A new health system for the 21st century.* Washington, DC: National Academy of Sciences.

Joint Commission. (2010). *Facts about patient safety.* Retrieved from http://www.jointcommission.org/AboutUs/Fact_Sheets/facts_patient

Kohn, K. T., Corrigan, J. M., & Donaldson, M. S. (Eds.). (2000). *To err is human: Building a safer health system.* Washington, DC: National Academy Press.

Licht, D. M., Polzella, D. J., & Boff, K. R. (n.d.). *Human factors, ergonomics and human factors engineering: An analysis of definitions.* Retrieved from http://www.dtic.mil/dticasd/docs/Human_Factors_Definitions.pdf

Maslow, A. (2009, November 11). *If the only tool you have is a hammer, you tend to see every problem as a nail.* Retrieved from http://blog.dreamthisday.com/2009/11/abraham-maslow-if-only-tool-you-have-is.html

Pizza, L., Goldfarb, N., & Nash, D. (2001). Crew resource management and its applications in medicine. In K. G. Shojania, B. W. Duncan, K. M. McDonald, & R. M. Wachter (Eds.), *Making health care safer* (Chapter 44). Retrieved from http://archive.ahrq.gov/clinic/ptsafety

Pronovost, P., Needham, D., Berenholtz, S., Sinopoli, D., Chu, H., Cosgrove, S., . . . Goeschel, C. (2006, December 28). An intervention to decrease catheter-related bloodstream infections in the ICU. *New England Journal of Medicine, 355,* 2725–2732.

Sackett, D. L., & Rosenberg, W. M. (1995). On the need for evidence-based medicine. *Journal of Public Health, 17,* P330–P334.

Senge, P. M. (1990). *The fifth discipline: The art & practice of the learning organization.* New York, NY: DoubleDay.

Wennberg, J., & Gittelsohn, A. (1982). Variations in medical care among small areas. *Scientific American, 246,* 120–134.

World Alliance for Patient Safety. (2008). *WHO surgical safety checklist and implementation manual.* Retrieved from http://www.who.int/patientsafety/safesurgery/ss_checklist/en/

2

Milestones of Hospital Accreditation and Patient Safety in the United States

*T*o understand the present and plan for the future, one must know the past. Until about 60 years ago, accreditation was not used as an external driver to promote quality and patient safety. In the early 1900s, most medical care was provided in the home. Hospitals had to overcome their image of being a house of death and/or a refuge for the poor—patients did not have a high degree of trust that safe care would be provided to them there.

With the industrial revolution, management in hospitals became focused on business practices and on the hospital as a scientific institution. The technology of this time centered on the development and use of medical records, refrigerators, laboratories, and sterilizers. During this time, nursing students provided most patient care, and the superintendents of hospitals were usually nurses (Margarete & Bigolow, 2007).

Certainly, a greater understanding of patient safety factors as well as the application of comprehensive accreditation standards now assists us in achieving better patient outcomes and focusing on continual improvement.

FOURTH CENTURY BC: HIPPOCRATIC OATH

Hippocrates provided a framework for ethical guidance and foundation for providing safe and effective health care to patients: "I will follow that system or regimen which according to my ability and judgment, I consider for the benefit of my patients and abstain from anything which is deleterious or mischievous."

Robbins (2005) has suggested that Hippocrates was an early decision theory and outcomes specialist, similar to Dr. Donald Berwick (past CEO for the Institute of Healthcare Improvement and currently the head of CMS). Robbins' reasoning is simple: Hippocrates believed that we should do something because it is the right thing to do, not merely "because it is in the black bag."

1818 TO 1865: IGNAZ PHILLIP SEMMELWEIS

Dr. Semmelweis was a Hungarian physician who introduced antiseptic prophylaxis into medicine. He observed that women in labor experienced high death rates when student doctors who examined them had not washed their hands after leaving the autopsy room. He ordered the students to wash their hands with chlorinated lime before examining the women, and the maternal death rate was reduced to approximately 1 percent within 2 years. Unfortunately, his work was not well received by the medical community of that time (Centers for Disease Control and Prevention [CDC], 2001).

1820 TO 1910: FLORENCE NIGHTINGALE

Florence Nightingale was one of the first leaders in patient safety. Her view as a nurse was that hospitals should help patients, not harm them. She used statistical analysis to measure results, and reduced preventable deaths in the Crimean War approximately from 42 percent to 2 percent (see Figure 2.1; McDonald, 2007). She was one of the first nursing professionals to advocate washing hands to fight infections. Nonetheless, she had to fight the medical community and go public with articles in *The Times* to gain support to implement sanitary patient care conditions (Simkin, n.d.).

Nightingale would be surprised to know that the medical community is not so different today. In 1999, Lucian Leape first noted in the Institute of Medicine's (IOM's) "To Err Is Human" report that between 44,000 and 98,000 deaths occur each year in U.S. hospitals. After the publication, he received much criticism and queries about the methodology

FIGURE 2.1

Florence Nightingale's diagram on the causes of mortality.

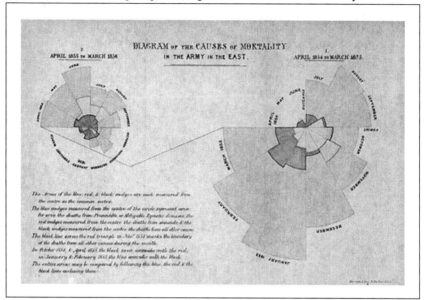

and accuracy in the numbers reported. He defended himself against his attackers publicly and stated, "Is it somehow better if the number is only 20,000 deaths? No, that's still horrible, and we need to fix it" (Leape, 2000).

1910: THE FLEXNER REPORT

The Flexner Report ushered in the first big wave of reform in medical education. Abraham Flexner was an educator whose career spanned more than 30 years at Rockefeller Institute for Medical Research in New York. After touring 150 medical schools in the United States and Canada, Flexner reported wide variation in the educational standards for physicians. His work led toward standardization of higher educational requirements for medical education (Flexner, 1910).

The second wave of potential change for reform in medical education occurred more recently, when the Lucian Leape Institute at the National Patient Safety Foundation (NPSF) released "Unmet needs: Teaching physicians to provide safe patient care" in 2010 stating that medical schools were inadequate at teaching physicians basic knowledge and skills required to provide safe care. The recommendations for medical schools centered on central themes: creating learning cultures, teaching patient safety as a basic science, intensive faculty development programs, so faculty can be role models for the change that needs to happen; with increased emphasis on personal attributes that reflect professionalism and concepts of patient safety as part of the admissions process (National Patient Safety Foundation [NPSF], 2010).

1869 TO 1940: ERNEST AMORY CODMAN

Dr. Codman was a Boston surgeon at Massachusetts General Hospital who wanted health care professionals such as physicians to learn from their medical errors. He advocated transparency and recorded diagnostic errors. His work was not well received by his peers, and Codman resigned from Massachusetts General Hospital. He then started his own hospital, which he called "The End Result Hospital." Codman reported the end results for patients who received care in his hospital, as seen in the following example:

> From 1911 to 1916, there were 337 patients discharged from his hospital with an average of one error made for every three patients. There were errors because of lack of knowledge or skill, surgical judgment, lack of care or equipment, and lack of diagnostic skill. (Neuhauser, 2007)

Codman's efforts for linking errors with end results earned him public ridicule and opposition; however, Codman became a member of the Society of Clinical Surgery, which led to creation of the American College of Surgeons in 1913. Codman was instrumental in the founding of the American College of Surgeons (ACS). ACS developed a hospital standardization program which later evolved into the Joint Commission. (Joint Commission, 2010).

It has now been almost 100 years since Codman's end result reports categorized medical errors. In March of 2009, two medical leaders, Dr. David Newman-Toker and Dr. Peter Pronovost, predicted that "diagnostic errors will be the next frontier for patient safety efforts" (Newman-Toker & Pronovost, 2009).

1919: AMERICAN COLLEGE OF SURGEONS MINIMUM STANDARDS FOR HOSPITALS

A document titled "American College of Surgeons Minimum Standards for Hospitals" in 1919 established the minimum requirements for hospital standards (see Figure 2.2). It contained only five

FIGURE 2.2

American College of Surgeons 1919: The minimum standard. (Reprinted with permission from the *Bulletin of the American College of Surgeons,* January 1920. Vol. IV, #3, p. 4, by American College of Surgeons.)

The Minimum Standard

1. That physicians and surgeons privileged to practice in the hospital be organized as a definite group or staff. Such organization has nothing to do with the question as to whether the hospital is "open" or "closed," nor need it affect the various existing types of staff organization. The word STAFF is here defined as the group of doctors who practice in the hospital inclusive of all groups such as the "regular staff," "the visiting staff," and the "associate staff."

2. That membership upon the staff be restricted to physicians and surgeons who are (a) full graduates of medicine in good standing and legally licensed to practice in their respective states or provinces; (b) competent in their respective fields and (c) worthy in character and in matters of professional ethics; that in this latter connection the practice of the division of fees, under any guise whatever, be prohibited.

3. That the staff initiate and, with the approval of the governing board of the hospital, adopt rules, regulations, and policies governing the professional work of the hospital; that these rules, regulations, and policies specifically provide:

   (a) That staff meetings be held at least once each month. (In large hospitals the departments may choose to meet separately.)

   (b) That the staff review and analyze at regular intervals their clinical experience in the various departments of the hospital, such as medicine, surgery, obstetrics, and the other specialties; the clinical records of patients, free and pay, to be the basis for such review and analyses.

4. That accurate and complete records be written for all patients and filed in an accessible manner in the hospital—a complete case record being one which includes identification data; complaint; personal and family history; history of present illness; physical examination; special examinations, such as consultations, clinical laboratory, X-ray and other examinations; provisional or working diagnosis; medical or surgical treatment; gross and microscopical pathological findings; progress notes; final diagnosis; condition on discharge; follow-up and, in case of death, autopsy findings.

5. That diagnostic and therapeutic facilities under competent supervision be available for the study, diagnosis, and treatment of patients, these to include, at least (a) a clinical laboratory providing chemical, bacteriological, serological, and pathological services; (b) an X-ray department providing radiographic and fluoroscopic services.

essential standards, three of which centered on the organization of the medical staff.

Today, the Joint Commission has more than 400 pages of standards that include organization of the medical staff, which require more than 150 elements of performance.

Be that as it may, when the first surveys of hospitals were conducted, the results were made public but the list of the actual hospitals was burned to prevent the press from reporting them to the public (Roberts, Coale, & Redman, 1987).

Finally, when the 1986 Health Care Financing Administration (HCFA) published the first hospital report cards with risk-adjusted Medicare mortality data, this report was not burned, but it created extensive controversy and criticism. From the controversy came the realization that wide variation in mortality outcomes existed between hospitals (Darby, 1998).

1953: JOINT COMMISSION ACCREDITATION OF HOSPITALS

The JCAH published the first set of required structure standards for hospitals. There were only 11 pages that contained governance expectations for the medical staff, which included some departmental standards. Now, the Joint Commission's manual is evolved from structure to process and outcome standards.

1964: JOSEPH M. JURAN PUBLISHES *MANAGERIAL BREAKTHROUGH*

Dr. Juran was one of the leaders who founded the quality movement and is credited with developing the Juran Trilogy of Quality Planning, Quality Control, and Quality Improvement. His quality concepts related to breakthrough have evolved into, what we know today as, Lean and Six Sigma (De Feo, n.d.).

Juran placed great emphasis on leadership and believed that quality was "freedom from errors that require doing work over again (rework) or that result in field failures, customer dissatisfaction, customer claims, and so on" (Juran & Godfrey, 1999).

Juran's emphasis on leadership and use of a learning cycle (Plan, Do, Study, Act) are used today as the foundation for implementing quality and patient safety programs.

1965: PASSAGE OF THE MEDICARE ACT

The Medicare Act tied Joint Commission standards to government requirements for Medicare Conditions of Participation (COPs) for Hospitals.

This meant that for a facility to be eligible to receive payment from Medicare or Medicaid, it must be certified, which requires having met the COPs set forth in federal regulations (Franko, 2002).

1970: JCAHO STANDARDS EVOLVE

JCAHO changed its standards to represent optimal and achievable levels of quality, instead of only minimally essential levels of quality. This transition occurred because most American hospitals were already meeting the minimum standards, Medicare had mandated compliance with more rigorous guidelines, and the techniques used to assess and improve quality had grown more sophisticated than in the past (Luce & Bindman, 1994).

1982: W. EDWARDS DEMING PUBLISHES *OUT OF THE CRISIS*

In addition to Juran, Dr. Deming (1986) was the other guru of quality who emerged in the 1950s. Like Juran, Deming placed great emphasis on leadership for quality. He felt that retrospective inspection was too late; quality needed to be built into the product. Deming modified and improved on the learning cycle process of Plan, Do, Study, Act, and he continually used the scientific method for improvement. His philosophy emphasized management accountability, appreciation of systems, and use of the learning cycle, which remain the foundation for effective quality and patient safety efforts today.

1984: CHARLES PERROW PUBLISHES *NORMAL ACCIDENTS: LIVING WITH HIGH-RISK TECHNOLOGIES*

Dr. Perrow provided a study of the aftermath of the Three Mile Island nuclear accident that occurred near Middletown, Pennsylvania, in 1979. Perrow felt that accidents were normal and inevitable. He defined two terms, *interactive complexity* and *loose/tight coupling*, which are used frequently today when health care organizations seek to become HROs (Perrow, 1984).

Interactive complexity is the degree to which we are unable to predict all of the ways in which things can go wrong. Interactive complexity acknowledges that every system holds the potential for unfamiliar or unplanned and unexpected sequences of events due to causes that are either not visible or not immediately comprehensible.

Loose/tight coupling refers to whether a system is tightly or loosely coupled. Tightly coupled refers to systems in which outcomes are tied to interdependencies and sequences of actions of events that one can control. Think of the operating room, where many processes are dependent on the performance of other processes that must be timed in a certain way to achieve a "safe" surgery. There is minimal or zero tolerance for errors. Tightly coupled systems enable small failures to cascade into complex interactions resulting in patient harm.

Loosely coupled systems, however, are those in which the sequence and precision of events are less influential on a system's outcome.

1985: ANESTHESIA PATIENT SAFETY FOUNDATION FORMED

The Anesthesia Patient Safety Foundation was the first medical specialty to champion patient safety as a specific focus. Speaking about the combined impact of all the initiatives of this foundation, R. K. Stoelting (n.d.) attributed a "10- to 20-fold reduction in mortality and catastrophic morbidity for healthy patients undergoing routine anesthetics, an evolution of which the entire profession can be justifiably proud."

1990: PETER SENGE PUBLISHES THE FIFTH DISCPLINE: THE ART AND PRACTICE OF THE LEARNING ORGANIZATION

Peter Senge (1990) built on Deming's work, particularly in appreciation for systems, Senge's five disciplnes of personal mastery, mental models, building a shared vision, team learning and system's thinking provide the foundation for the learning organization. Senge's work is widely used for developing learning organizations and implementing effective quality and patient safety programs.

1990: JAMES REASON PUBLISHES *HUMAN ERROR*

Dr. Reason (1990), formerly a professor of psychology at the University of Manchester, England, developed an expertise in the causes of human error. He defined two types of errors: slips and lapses and mistakes. Slips and lapses occur when a person does an action he or she did not intend to do. They are apt to occur during routine activities that have been performed many times before and are performed when our brain is on autopilot. Fatigue, interruptions, and time pressures trigger these types of errors. A lapse results from a failure of memory.

Mistakes are made as a result of following through with a wrong plan of action. Mistakes involve misinterpretation of the problem, a lack of knowledge, or common but ineffective patterns of thought.

It is important to know which types of errors occur, because the preventive interventions are different depending on the type of error made. For a long time, the medical community just blamed, trained, and shamed.

Reason (2000) is also known for his "Swiss Cheese" model of human error, which says that when organizational failures become lined up in perfect sequence and the holes are perfectly aligned, accidents happen. This means that errors pass through a series of barriers that permit a path for an accident opportunity. His model is widely used today when analysis of adverse events is performed.

1991: NEW ENGLAND JOURNAL OF MEDICINE PUBLISHES THE *HARVARD MEDICAL PRACTICE STUDY*

In the *Harvard Medical Practice Study*, Brennan et al. (1991) described the incidence of adverse events as "injuries caused by medical management, and of the subgroup of such injuries that resulted from negligent or substandard care."

The study estimated that adverse events occurred in 3.7 percent of all hospitalizations: 27.6 percent of the adverse events were because of negligence, 2.6 percent caused permanently disabling injuries, and 13.6 percent resulted in death. This report, when first published, was surrounded with controversy, and some of the medical community questioned the accuracy of the numbers.

1992: JCAHO STARTS TO TRANSITION FROM DEPARTMENTAL STANDARDS TO IMPORTANT ORGANIZATIONAL FUNCTIONS

The Joint Commission started to emphasize performance-based standards in 1992. To carry out these functions effectively required a multidisciplinary team approach (Appel, 1991). Team approaches are essential when implementing patient safety efforts.

1994: BETSY LEHMAN DIES FROM AN OVERDOSE

Betsy Lehman, a respected health care journalist, died from an accidental overdose of chemotherapy while being cared for at the Dana-Farber Cancer Institute. The incident was highly publicized and drew national attention. One of the outcomes of this tragedy was that the Dana-Farber Cancer Institute redoubled its efforts to become one of the leaders in implementing patient safety practices (Dana-Farber Cancer Institute, n.d.).

1996: INSTITUTE OF MEDICINE PUBLISHES *NURSING STAFF IN HOSPITALS AND NURSING HOMES: IS IT ADEQUATE?*

The Committee on the Adequacy of Nurse Staffing in Hospitals and Nursing Homes formed by the IOM concluded that, even though the literature on registered nurses' impact on mortality is considerable, not enough research exists in the areas of the effects of structural measures, such as specific staffing ratios.

The committee recommended that there should be "a high priority given to obtaining empirical evidence that permits one to draw conclusions about the relationships of quality of inpatient care and staffing levels and mix" (IOM, 1996).

1996: THE SENTINEL EVENT POLICY IS INITIATED BY THE JOINT COMMISSION

The Joint Commission defines a Sentinel Event (SE) as "an unexpected occurrence involving death or serious physical or psychological injury. . . . Serious injury specifically includes loss of limb or function" (n.d.-a).

When a SE occurs, the health care organization is required to perform a credible RCA, implement improvements to reduce the risk, and monitor the effectiveness of the improvements. The Joint Commission emphasized that analysis of the system, not the provider, was essential for risk reduction.

1998: THE QUALITY INTERAGENCY COORDINATION TASK FORCE

The Quality Interagency Coordination Task Force (QuIC) was established in accordance with President Clinton's directive. Its purpose was to ensure that all federal agencies involved in "purchasing, providing, studying, or regulating health care services were working in a coordinated manner toward the common goal of improving quality care" (QuIC, n.d.). Work groups have been established to identify and work on projects within identified topic areas, and a major focus has been identifying ways in which to address medical errors.

1999: JCAHO'S MISSION STATEMENT CHANGES

The Joint Commission added the words "continuously" and "safety" to its mission statement, so it now reads: "To continuously improve the safety and quality of health care" (2010). With this change, patient safety became integrated within the Joint Commission's mission.

2000: NATIONAL QUALITY FORUM BECOMES FULLY OPERATIONAL

The National Quality Forum (NQF) is a nonprofit organization whose aim is to improve the health of all Americans by setting national priorities, developing national consensus standards, and promoting national goals through education and outreach programs (NQF, n.d.).

2000: THE INSTITUTE OF MEDICINE PUBLISHES *TO ERR IS HUMAN: BUILDING A SAFER HEALTH SYSTEM*

To Err Is Human: Building a Safer Health System extrapolated the results from previous studies to infer that at least 44,000 to 98,000 Americans died each year as a result of medical errors. Four recommendations were made:

1. Enhance the knowledge base about safety by establishing a national focus to create leadership, research tools, and protocols.
2. Make sure the system continues to be made safer for patients by identifying and learning from errors through immediate and strong mandatory reporting efforts as well as the encouragement of voluntary efforts.
3. Raise performance standards and expectations for improvements in safety through the actions of oversight organizations, professional groups, and group purchasers of health care.
4. Implement safety systems in health care organizations to ensure safe practices at the delivery level. This is the ultimate goal for all of the recommendations.

This publication acted as a catalyst for implementing changes needed for patient safety (Kohn, Corrigan, & Donaldson, 2000).

2001: THE INSTITUTE OF MEDICINE PUBLISHES *THE RECOMMENDATIONS MADE BY THE COMMITTEE ON THE QUALITY OF HEALTH CARE IN AMERICA IN CROSSING THE QUALITY CHASM: A NEW HEALTH SYSTEM FOR THE TWENTY-FIRST CENTURY*

This second report followed *To Err is Human* and provided the national agenda for action for redesigning the twenty-first–century health care system. The major recommendations were as follows:

- A shared agenda of six aims for improvement that can raise the quality of care to unprecedented levels
- Adoption of a new set of principles to guide the redesign of care processes

- Identification by the Department of Health and Human Services (DHHS) of a set of priority conditions on which to focus initial efforts and provide resources to stimulate innovation and initiate the change process
- Design and implementation by health care organizations of more effective organizational support processes to make change in the delivery of care possible
- Creation of an environment that fosters and rewards improvement on the part of purchasers, regulators, health professions, educational institutions, and the DHHS.

2001: UNITED STATES CONGRESS INCREASES AGENCY FOR HEALTHCARE RESEARCH AND QUALITY'S PATIENT SAFETY RESEARCH BUDGET

The AHRQ's budget rose substantially, from US$20 million to US$50 million for 2001. This represented the single largest investment the federal government had ever made to fight medical errors (Keyes et al., 2005).

2001: THE TERM *NEVER EVENT* IS INTRODUCED

Ken Kizer, former CEO of NQF, referred to adverse events that should never occur, such as wrong-site surgery, as *never events* (AHRQ, n.d.). Later (see entry for 2008), Medicare created a list of nonpayable adverse events, which were based on this concept. The principle is that consumers and insurers should not have to pay when preventable harm is done while under the care of the provider.

2001: CENTRAL LINES ARE TACKLED BY PETER PRONOVOST

Critical care specialist at Johns Hopkins Hospital, Dr. Peter Pronovost, tackled central line infections with a simple checklist and measured the results for a year afterward; the 10-day line infection rate "went from eleven percent to zero" (Gawande, 2007). No longer would these types of infections be accepted within a threshold range—zero is the acceptable number.

2002: NQF ENDORSES A LIST OF SERIOUS REPORTABLE EVENTS

The NQF announced a list of serious reportable events (SREs), which would increase public accountability and consumer access to critical information about health care performance (NQF, 2008). The list of SREs provided a consensus on the most egregious medical errors for which the health care system should be held accountable.

Examples include surgery performed on the wrong body part or patient, retention of a foreign object after surgery, or infants discharged to the wrong person. This list was built on *never event* concepts.

2003: FIRST SET OF NATIONAL PATIENT SAFETY GOALS BECOME EFFECTIVE IN JANUARY

National Patient Safety Goals (NPSGs) were initiated to assist accredited organizations to address specific areas of concern regarding patient safety. The goals were developed by the Patient Safety Advisory Group working with Joint Commission staff who performed a systematic literature review as well as a review of available databases prior to deciding on the selection of the first NPSGs (Joint Commission, n.d.-b). Health care organizations surveyed by the Joint Commission had to demonstrate compliance with meeting the NPSGs as part of their survey process.

2003: NATIONAL QUALITY FORUM PUBLISHES FIRST SET OF 30 NATIONAL SAFE PRACTICES

National safe practices were researched and felt to have great potential for reducing adverse events (Kizer & Blum, n.d.). This was the first national attention focused on patient safety practices thought to mitigate adverse events in health care organizations.

2004: AHRQ RELEASES THE HOSPITAL SURVEY ON PATIENT SAFETY CULTURE

The Hospital Survey on Patient Safety Culture (AHRQ, 2004) consisted of a staff survey designed to assist hospitals to assess their culture of safety in their organizations. Since its creation in 2004, the survey has spread internationally and the AHRQ site maintains a database containing the results (AHRQ, n.d.). Culture is acknowledged as a key driver for patient safety efforts. The Joint Commission now requires an assessment of the culture of safety as part of its standards.

2004: OFFICE OF THE NATIONAL COORDINATOR FOR HEALTH CARE INFORMATION TECHNOLOGY IS CREATED

The Office of the National Coordinator for Health Care Information Technology (ONC) was charged with coordination of nationwide efforts to develop a nationwide infrastructure for electronic use and exchange of information. Computer databases are essential for patient safety efforts. This was the nationwide effort to computerize health care (ONC, n.d.).

2004: "100,000 LIVES CAMPAIGN" IS INITIATED AS A NATIONAL MOVEMENT BY THE INSTITUTE FOR HEALTHCARE IMPROVEMENT

The goal of the "100,000 Lives Campaign" was to significantly reduce morbidity and mortality in American health care.

The initial goals included deployment of rapid response teams, delivering reliable, evidence-based care for acute myocardial infarction, preventing adverse drug events (ADEs) through medication reconciliation, preventing central line infections, preventing surgical-site infections, and preventing ventilator-associated pneumonia. "Some is not a number, soon is not a time: the number is 100,000; the time is NOW" (Wachter and Provonost, 2006).

2004 JULY: JOINT COMMISSION INITIATES THE UNIVERSAL PROTOCOL

Wrong site, wrong procedure, wrong person surgery adverse events were labeled as SEs by the Joint Commission, and the universal protocol as a patient safety goal was initiated as a response to receiving continuing reports of this occurrence. The universal protocol, which consists of a standardized set of steps to follow, was developed as a solution to prevent these adverse events from reoccurring (Joint Commission, n.d.-c).

2005: PATIENT SAFETY AND QUALITY IMPROVEMENT ACT (PUBLIC LAW 109 TO 141) IS PASSED

The Patient Safety and Quality Improvement Act (PSQIA) created Patient Safety Organizations (PSOs) to collect, aggregate, and analyze confidential information reported by health care providers. This act provided federal legal privilege and confidentiality protections to information provided regarding medical errors. It was hoped that this legislation would assist disclosure and reporting efforts of medical errors. This enhanced reporting would assist with aggregation of information and subsequent learning by the health care systems to reduce future risks (Fasset, 2006).

2008: CENTERS FOR MEDICARE/MEDICAID DENIES PAYMENT FOR CERTAIN ADVERSE EVENTS

Medicare no longer pays the extra cost of treating the following categories of conditions that occur while the patient is in the hospital:

> Pressure ulcer stages III and IV, falls and trauma, surgical-site infection after bariatric surgery for obesity, certain orthopedic procedures and bypass surgery (mediastinitis), vascular-catheter-associated infection, catheter-associated urinary tract infection, administration of incompatible blood, air embolism, and foreign object unintentionally retained after surgery. (CMS, 2008)

These *never events* will not receive reimbursement, a condition that provides an external incentive for health care organizations to take actions to prevent these types of events.

2009: CENTER FOR TRANSFORMING HEALTH CARE IS STARTED

The Joint Commission collaborates with volunteer hospitals and health systems across the United States and launches the *Center for Transforming Healthcare*. One of the first projects undertaken was Hand Hygiene. The goal of this project was to make care safer by providing increased reliability in adherence to hand-hygiene protocols (Joint Commission, 2009). The center uses Robust Improvement Processes such as Lean or Six Sigma to find evidence-based solutions to share with health care organizations that can match their unique problems to corresponding solutions.

CONCLUSIONS

Accreditation and patient safety have a long history that continues to evolve. Both initiatives involved pioneers who suffered public ridicule and controversy by the medical community when their information was first presented regarding adverse outcomes. Increasingly, accreditation is integrating patient safety concepts into the accreditation process for health care systems.

REFERENCES

Agency for Healthcare Research and Quality. (2004). *Hospital survey on patient safety culture.* Retrieved 14 October, 2011 from http://www.ahrq.gov/qual/patientsafetyculture/hospsurvindex.htm

Agency for Healthcare Research and Quality. (n.d.). *Patient safety primer: Never events.* Retrieved April 24, 2010, from http://www.psnet.ahrq.gov/primer.aspx?primerID=3

Appel, F. (1991). From quality assurance to quality improvement: The Joint Commission and the new quality paradigm. *Journal of Quality Assurance, 13*(5), 26–29.

Berwick, D. (n.d.). *Overview of the 100,000 lives campaign.* Retrieved April 24, 2010, from http://www.ihi.org/IHI/Programs/Campaign/100kCampaignOverviewArchive.htm

Brennan, T. A., Leape, L. L., Laird, N. M., Hebert, L., Localio, A. R., Lawthers, A. G., . . . Hiatt, H. H. (1991). Incidence of adverse events and negligence in hospitalized patients. Results of the Harvard Practice Study I. *New England Journal of Medicine, 324*(6), 370–376.

Centers for Disease Control and Prevention. (2001). Ignaz Philipp Semmelweis (1818–65; about the cover). *Emerging Infectious Diseases, 7*(2). Retrieved April 23, 2010, from http://www.cdc.gov/ncidod/eid/vol7no2/cover.htm#cit

CMS (2010). *Hospital-acquired conditions (HAC) and Present on Admission Indicator Reporting.* Retrieved 15 October, 2011, from http://www.cms.gov/HospitalAcqCond/downloads/HACFactsheet.pdf

Dana-Farber Cancer Institute. (n.d.). *Dana-Farber's patient safety journey.* Retrieved April 24, 2010, from http://www.dana-farber.org/Adult-Care/Treatment-and-Support/Care-Quality-and-Safety/Patient-Safety-Journey.aspx

Darby, M. (1998). *Health care quality: From data to accountability.* Washington, DC: The George Washington University. Retrieved September 6, 2010, from http://www.nhpf.org/library/background-papers/BP_100_HCData_2-98.pdf

De Feo, J. A. (n.d.). *Joseph M. Juran 1904–2008.* Retrieved April 24, 2010, from http://www.juran.com/about_juran_institute_our_founder.html

Deming, W. E. (1986). *Out of the crisis.* Cambridge, UK: Cambridge University Press.

Fasset, W. E. (2006). *Patient Safety and Quality Improvement Act of 2005.* Retrieved September 6, 2010, from http://www.medscape.com/viewarticle/532889

Flexner, A. (1910). *Medical education in the United States and Canada: Bulletin Number Four (The Flexner Report): The Carnegie Foundation for the Advancement of Teaching.* Retrieved April 15, 2010, from http://www.carnegiefoundation.org/publications/medical-education-united-states-and-canada-bulletin-number-four-flexner-report-0

Franko, F. P. (2002). *The important role of Joint Commission-health policy issues-Joint Commission accreditation of health care organizations.* Retrieved April 15, 2010, from http://findarticles.com/p/search/?qt=important+role+of+joint+commission+health+policy+issues

Gawande, A. (2007). The checklist. *The New Yorker.* Retrieved April 24, 2010, from http://www.newyorker.com/reporting/2007/12/10/071210fa_fact_gawande

Institute of Medicine. (1996). *Nursing staff in hospitals and nursing homes: Is it adequate?* Washington, DC: National Academy Press.

Institute of Medicine. (2001). *Crossing the quality chasm: A new health system for the 21st century.* Washington, DC: National Academy Press.

Joint Commission. (2009). *Joint Commission Center for Transforming Healthcare takes aim at patient safety failures.* Retrieved September 6, 2010, from http://www.jointcommission.org/NewsRoom/NewsReleases/cth_nr_9_10_09.htm

Joint Commission. (2010). *The Joint Commission history.* Retrieved January 10, 2011, from http://www.jointcommission.org/the_joint_commission_history/

Joint Commission. (n.d.-a). *Sentinel event.* Retrieved September 5, 2010, from http://www.jointcommission.org/SentinelEvents/

Joint Commission. (n.d.-b). *National patient safety goals.* Retrieved April, 19, from http://www.jointcommission.org/PatientSafety/NationalPatientSafetyGoals/

Joint Commission. (n.d.-c). *Facts about the universal protocol.* Retrieved January 1, 2011, from http://www.jointcommission.org/facts_about_the_universal_protocol

Juran, J. M., & Godfrey, A. B. (1999). *Juran's quality handbook* (5th ed.). New York, NY: McGraw-Hill.

Keyes, M. A., Ortiz, E., Queenan, D., Hughes, R., Chesley, F., & Hogan, E. M. (2005). *A strategic approach for funding research: The Agency for Healthcare Research and Quality's Patient Safety Initiative 2000–2004.* Retrieved April 24, 2010, from http://www.ncbi.nlm.nih.gov/bookshelf/br.fcgi? book=aps4&part=A6179

Kizer, K. W., & Blum, L. N. (n.d.). *Safe practices for better health care.* Retrieved April 24, 2010, from http://www.ncbi.nlm.nih.gov/bookshelf/br.fcgi? book=aps4&part=A6294

Kohn, L. T., Corrigan, J. M., & Donaldson, M. S. (Eds.). (2000). *To err is human: Building a safer health system.* Washington, DC: National Academy Press.

Leape, L. (2000). Institute of Medicine medical errors figures are not exaggerated. *Journal of American Medical Association, 284,* 95–97.

Luce, J. M., & Bindman, A. B. (1994). *A brief history of health care quality assessment and improvement in the United States.* Retrieved April 15, 2010, from http://www.ncbi.nlm.nih.gov/pmc/articles/PMC1022402/pdf/west jmed00067-0065.pdf

Margarete, A., & Bigolow, B. (2007). *Hospital administration in the early 1900's: Visions for the future and the reality of daily practice.* Retrieved September 6, 2010, from http://www.entrepreneur.com/tradejournals/ article/158907311_3.htm

McDonald, L. (2007). Florence Nightingale and European wars: From the Crimean to the Franco_Prussian War. *Leidschrift Historisch Tijdscrift.* Retrieved April 15, 2010, from http://www.uoguelph.ca/~cwfn/whats new/franco.html

National Patient Safety Foundation (NPSF) (2010). Report of the Lucian Leape Institute Roundtable on reforming medical education. *Unmet needs: Teaching physicians to provide safe patient care.* Retrieved 16 October, 2011, from http://www.npsf.org/download/LLI-Unmet-Needs-Report.pdf

National Quality Forum. (2008). *Serious reportable events.* Retrieved April 24, 2010, from http://www.qualityforum.org/Publications/2008/ 10/Serious_Reportable_Events.aspx

National Quality Forum. (n.d.). Retrieved September 5, 2010, from http:// www.qualityforum.org/

Neuhauser, D. (2007). Heroes and martyrs of quality and patient safety: Ernest Amory Codman MD. *Quality and Safety in Health Care.* Retrieved April 1 5, 2010, from http://qshc.bmj.com/content/11/1/104.full

Newman-Toker, D. E., & Pronovost, P. J. (2009). Diagnostic errors-the next frontier for patient safety. *Journal of American Medical Association, 301*(10), 1060–1062.

The Office of the National Coordinator for Health Information Technology. (n.d.). Retrieved April 24, 2010, from http://healthit.hhs.gov/portal/server.pt?open=512&objID=1200&mode=2

Perrow, C. (1984). *Normal accidents: Living with high-risk technologies.* New York, NY: Basic Books.

QuIC. (n.d.). *Quality Interagency Coordination (QuIC) Task Force.* Retrieved April 24, 2010, from http://www.quic.gov/

Reason, J. (1990). *Human error.* New York, NY: Cambridge University Press.

Reason, J. (2000). *Human error: models and management.* Retrieved 15 October, 2011, from http://www.bmj.com/content/320/7237/768.full

Robbins, D. A. (2005). Health advice from the 4th century BC: Ethics toolbox. *Patient Safety & Quality Healthcare.* Retrieved April 23, 2010, from http://www.psqh.com/novdec05/ethics.html

Roberts, J. S., Coale, J. G., & Redman, R. R. (1987). A history of the Joint Commission on accreditation of hospitals. Special communication. *Journal of American Medical Association, 258*(7), 936–940.

Senge, P. M. (1990). *The fifth discipline: The art & practice of the learning organization.* New York, NY: Double Day.

Simkin, J. (n.d.) *Spartacus educational.* Retrieved September 5, 2010, from http://www.spartacus.schoolnet.co.uk/REnightingale.htm

Stoelting, R. K. (n.d.). *Anesthesia patient safety foundation. APSF history overview: A brief history of APSF.* Retrieved April 23, 2010, from http://www.apsf.org/about_history.php

Wachter, R. M., Provonost, P. J. (2006). *The 100,000 lives campagin: a scientific and policy review.* Retrieved 14 October, 2011, from http://health caredisclosure.org/docs/files/100KLivesCampaign062408.pdf

3

A Global View of Patient Safety and Accreditation

UNITED STATES

The mission of the Office of Inspector General (OIG) is to "protect the integrity of DHHS programs, as well as the health and welfare of the beneficiaries of those programs" (OIG, n.d.).

According to PR Newswire (2010), the OIG reported that one in seven Medicare patients was harmed by the care they received in a hospital. The study was based on a nationally representative sample of 780 Medicare patients during the month of October 2008. During that month, 134,000 Medicare patients experienced harm while under their provider's care in a hospital. The OIG calculated that the medical harm cost an additional US$324 million in hospital care. Annualized, this cost for medical harm was estimated to be US$4.4 billion.

Schoen and Colleagues' article in *The Commonwealth Fund* (2005) assessed health care access, safety, and care coordination in Australia, New Zealand, Canada, the United Kingdom, and the United States and reported that the United States has the highest rate of any country for patients who experience medical, medication, or test errors.

One-third of Americans with health problems reported experiencing medical mistakes, medication errors, or inaccurate or delayed lab results; this was the highest rate reported among the six nations surveyed.

The United States was the highest in error rates and inefficient coordination of care. In addition, high out-of-pocket costs resulted in patients' bypassing necessary medical care simply because they could not afford it. In fact, one-half of adults with health problems in the United States stated that they did not go to a doctor when sick, did not follow through with recommended treatment, or did not obtain the needed medications prescribed because of the cost. This means that Americans put themselves at risk for premature, preventable deaths because of delaying necessary diagnostic tests with subsequent treatments.

CANADA

Gagnon (2004) reported that Canada's Institute for Health Information's (CIHI) annual report found that medical errors in Canada are common and that there are significant regional disparities in how the health care system performs.

Almost one out of every four Canadians said that either they or a family member experienced a preventable, adverse event in 2003. This equates to approximately 5.2 million people. The adverse events reported ranged from patients receiving the wrong dosage or wrong type of medication to having foreign objects left in their body after surgery.

Also within CIHI's annual report, Canada reported significant variation in performance in some health performance indicators. In Nova Scotia, 24.2 percent of patients who experienced a stroke died in the hospital within 30 days, whereas in Alberta, 15.5 percent of the patients who experienced a stroke died.

Baker et al. (2004) estimated the incidence of adverse events to be 7.5 percent per 100 hospital admissions, and 36.9 percent of these were judged as preventable in acute care hospitals in Canada. When these data are extrapolated for the 2.5 million annual hospital admissions in Canada in similar type hospitals, this translates into approximately 185,000 adverse events of which 70,000 are potentially preventable.

In response to the issues generated by potentially avoidable adverse events, the Canadian Patient Safety Institute (CPSI) was established in 2003. It is an independent and nonprofit corporation that works collaboratively with health providers and organizations, regulatory bodies, and governments with the aim of building and advancing a safer health care system for Canadians. CPSI's role is to "provide a leadership role with respect to patient safety issues in the context of improving health care quality." CPSI has advanced patient safety initiatives through supporting and coordinating key initiatives to ensure that evidence-based information is disseminated across the health care continuum. Examples of patient safety initiatives include the Hand Hygiene Campaign, Canadian Patient Safety Week, and the Safer Healthcare Now Campaign, which is patterned after the Institute of Healthcare Improvement's (IHI's) 1,000 Lives Campaign (CPSI, n.d.).

UNITED KINGDOM

The United Kingdom reported in 2004 that within the National Health Service (NHS), one in 10 patients admitted, experienced a medical error. The medical accidents and errors contributed to 72,000 deaths, of which, 40,000 deaths were cited as being the direct result of medical accidents and errors. The NHS costs associated with medical errors were estimated at £2 billion just for increased hospital stays.

Along with that, an independent audit reported that fewer than one-third of the estimated 900,000 annual mistakes were properly reported (Woolcock & Henderson, 2004).

The National Patient Safety Agency (NPSA) was established in 2001 for England and Wales with the aim of raising awareness of patient safety issues and developing a national system of incident reporting. This agency was created to make patient safety a top priority for the NHS staff and boards of NHS management. NPSA comprises the National Reporting and Learning Service, the National Clinical Assessment Service, and the National Research Ethics Service. Through the three divisions, they cover the UK health service to "lead and contribute to improved, safe patient care by informing, supporting and influencing organizations and people working in the health sector." Accomplishments of NPSA in 2009 included improved reporting methods, increased risk awareness of the scale and risk of harm across England and Wales, and support for the Patient Safety First Campaign in England and 1,000 Lives Campaign in Wales (NPSA, 2010).

AUSTRALIA

In Ocober of 2008, the Australian news reported that it has been widely accepted for the past 10 years that approximately 1 in 10 Australian patients experienced a medical error during their hospital stay ("Don't Put Faith", 2008).

Lorraine Long founded the Medical Error Action Group in response to the death of her mother, June Long, in 1994, 14 hours after she entered a hospital following an asthma attack. The death was later attributed to medical errors. The group was formed to provide education to the public on how to seek truth when medical errors occur in hospitals.

According to the Medical Error Action Group, deaths caused by medical error in Australian hospitals kill 18,000 Australians and harm an estimated 330,000 persons every year, making medical error the leading cause of death and injury (Medical Error Action Group, 2008).

The Australian Patient Safety Foundation (APSF) is a nonprofit and independent entity that is dedicated to the advancement of patient safety. They have been in existence since 1988 and work with other agencies, commonwealth and state governments, researchers, academic institutions, health care professionals, and consumers at the national and the international levels. The foundation's aim is to improve outcomes for patients. In 2009 and 2010, the APSF continued training undergraduate and postgraduate health care providers in South Australia, published relevant research articles and reports, and provided technical and analytical support to users of incident reporting software (APSF, n.d.).

JAPAN

The IV team (2008) cited an article in *Japan's Mainichi Daily News* that the annual near-miss number for medical errors in Japan was 200,000 in 2007 and that more than 3,000 of these events had the potential for death. The survey conducted by the Japan Council for Quality Health Care also reported that greater than 25 percent of the near-miss cases involved prescription errors. Nurses were identified as the primary persons involved in near misses 73 percent of the time. Causes of mistakes related to medications involved mistakes in patient identification, mistakes in the type or dose of drug, and mistakes in setting correct rates for intravenous drips (IV Team, 2008).

Japan's Ministry of Health, Labor, and Welfare established an adverse event reporting system in 2007 that imposed mandatory reporting with legal punishment for the physician for noncompliance. The report was also allowed to be used in civil law suits, criminal prosecutions along with administrative sanctions. This created increased incidents of defensive medicine, especially in obstetrics and emergency medicine. There was one worst case cited, where one unfortunate patient was refused by 27 hospitals. This report concluded that

other countries may wish to learn from Japan's combined mandatory and accountability reporting system and the unintended results
that it achieved when medical practitioners feared reporting events
(Soichero, Masahiro, & Yoshinori, 2009).

WORLD HEALTH ORGANIZATION'S ROLE IN PATIENT SAFETY

The WHO is the international entity responsible for directing and
coordinating international health that is within the purview of the
United Nations. WHO has experts who produce standards and guidelines to assist countries with addressing their public health issues.

Numerous studies on health research are carried out and published. WHO is the entity that allows governments across the world
to collaborate to implement actions that are ultimately designed to
improve people's well-being.

WHO has many partners that include but are not limited to UN
agencies, nongovernmental organizations, WHO collaborating centers,
and the private sector. The WHO continually scans the environment to
seek and acquire new partnerships that will enhance achievement of
their goals (WHO, n.d.-a).

The WHO believes that both quality and patient safety are
essential attributes for providing good health services. In 2006, the
WHO endorsed a systematic process whereby a health care system
should seek to make improvements in their dimensions of quality.
The six dimensions noted by WHO are identical to those established
by the IOM:

Safe: delivering health care that minimizes risks and harm to service users

Effective: delivering health care that is adherent to an evidence base
and results in improved health outcomes for individuals and communities, based on need

Efficient: delivering health care in a manner that maximizes resource
use and avoids waste

Accessible: delivering health care that is timely, geographically reasonable, and provided in a setting where skills and resources are
appropriate to medical need

Acceptable/patient-centered: delivering health care that takes into
account the preferences and aspirations of individual service users
and the cultures of their communities

Equitable: delivering health care that does not vary in quality because of personal characteristics such as gender, race, ethnicity, geographical location, or socioeconomic status

In 2004, WHO initiated a worldwide patient safety program. This was in response to the World Health Assembly Resolutions in 2002 in which the WHO and member states were requested to pay utmost attention to the importance of patient safety as a global health care concern.

Since then, the World Alliance for Patient Safety was formed in 2004 with global leaders from around the world, with the aim to "First, do no harm." The goal of this aim was to reduce the number of adverse health and social consequences that were a direct result of unsafe health care (WHO, n.d.-b). Areas of concern included hand hygiene, unsafe injection practices, problems with surgical safety, and preventable heath care–associated infection (HAI). The six action areas embarked on in 2005 to 2006 were the following:

Clean care is safer care: a campaign to reduce HAI

Engagement of patients and consumers through benchmarks such as the Joint Commission's *Speak up for Patient Safety Program*

Development of centralized collection of patient safety taxonomy data, which has the capacity for comparisons across reporting systems

Sponsorship and encouragement of research in the field of patient safety

Development of solutions that reduce the risk of health care and improve its safety

Development of ways to improve patient safety through sharing lessons learned, use of alerts, and dissemination of information

The website *www.who.int/patientsafety* was developed to support international communication in this regard (WHO, 2004).

In 2009, WHO published a paper (Flin, Winter, Sarac, & Raduma, 2009). This report provided a basic description of the major topic areas relating to human factors relevant to patient safety. The 10 topic areas that were covered were organizational culture, managerial leadership, communication, teamwork, team leadership, situation awareness, decision making, stress, fatigue, and work environment. This is valuable information as health care organizations continue to work on leadership development and cultures. The following list shows a sampling of websites of useful leadership questionnaires:

www.mindgarden.com—measures the dimensions of leadership (transformational, transactional, laissez-faire, with outcomes of leadership such as effort, effectiveness and satisfaction)

www.leadershipchallenge.com—measures the five key leadership practices and is available in a number of languages for a fee

www.nhsleadershipqualities.nhs.uk—NHS Leadership Qualities Framework (LQF) can also be used for upward peer appraisal. The three categories of LQF are setting direction, personal qualities, and delivering service

Tools that are free of charge include the following:

www.eimicrosites.org/heartsandminds—provides the tool free for self- and upward appraisal of manager's safety leadership

www.ahrq.gov/qual/patientsafetyculture/—free questionnaire that measures 12 dimensions for both clinical and nonclinical staff, at the unit and management levels in hospitals; widely used globally, different versions available for different settings (e.g., nursing homes)

GLOBAL VIEW OF HOSPITAL ACCREDITATION

According to Shaw (2004), an extensive study was carried out in 2000 and reported that accreditation programs were rapidly increasing around the world, especially in South America and Europe. Only eight accreditation programs existed prior to 1991, but they nearly tripled within the next 10 years. More than 50 percent of the accreditation programs initiated since 1990 are in Europe.

Rather than rely on agendas for voluntary self-development, governments are increasingly using accreditation as a method to regulate and build public accountability.

The U.S. hospital accreditation program was established in 1951, followed by Canada in 1958, Australia in 1974, Taiwan in 1986, New Zealand in 1989, and the United Kingdom in 1990.

The number of accreditation programs doubled in 1990 to 1995 and then more than doubled again in the following 5 years. Global accreditation is growing rapidly and includes the integration of patient safety efforts.

In addition to hospitals adhering to a set of standards set by accrediting agencies, those agencies themselves must also meet a set of standards to ensure that they are doing the right thing. The body that accredits the accreditors is the International Society for Quality in Health Care (ISQua). The Joint Commission, Canada, and Australia, three major players in the global market for accreditation, are all ISQua accredited.

Because accreditation is critical to implement patient safety efforts, I interviewed three global leaders within these organizations to get their take on aspects of patient safety. The following interviews include information these leaders provided regarding their accreditation programs.

Joint Commission

Interview with Paul Schyve, MD, Senior Vice President, Joint Commission, August 5, 2010.

Q: Dr. Schyve, does Joint Commission have any plans to include Quality of Worklife (QWL) as part of the measures for organizational culture?

A: That is an interesting question. We have a Patient Safety Advisory Group that has on its list of potential topics for SE Alerts the issue of worker fatigue, which is an important aspect of QWL.

The topic of worker fatigue would fall under a potential SE Alert or something like it, we are considering creating another type of notice such as a "Patient Safety Advisory" for topics that don't necessarily qualify as SE Alert material. We would present what is known about the problem and some proposed solutions for it.

Another Joint Commission notice that comes to mind is our SE Alert and associated leadership standards on eliminating intimidating (or "disruptive") behaviors, which I would put into the QWL domain as well. The term *disruptive* may be a misnomer; the Joint Commission borrowed that label from others in the fields who were already using it.

The reason "disruptive" may be a misnomer is that there are times when disruptive behavior is desirable, such as occurs in the time-out step identified in the universal protocol for preventing wrong procedure, including wrong site and wrong person procedures. The time-out is a deliberate action that is *intended* to be disruptive so that the team takes a pause from their actions and ensures patient safety is maintained. This is analogous to stopping a train to make sure it is on the right track before moving forward.

The SE Alert on intimidating behavior was issued to stop the kind of behaviors that hinder people from speaking up and talking about actual or potential patient safety risks—intimidating behaviors that interfere with a patient safety culture. Intimidating behavior, unlike disruptive behavior, is *never* desirable.

The Medical Staff standard MS.01.01.01 is also related to a culture of safety. It was a multiyear project to rewrite this standard about the relationship between the governing body and the medical staff in a hospital. The importance of this standard is best understood in the context of the leadership standards that require that the governing body, the CEO and other senior leaders, and the medical staff work *collaboratively* to assume accountability for developing and maintaining a culture of patient safety.

To work collaboratively, both the medical staff and the governing body must agree on the parameters and the processes for their working together in the interest of the quality and safety of patient care. These agreements are codified in the medical staff bylaws—this is the focus of MS.01.01.01.

Q: Joint Commission requires one proactive risk assessment. Will Lean and/or Six Sigma be encouraged in the future as Robust Process Improvement (RPI) methods to increase reliability?

A: Our current requirement is for only one proactive risk assessment every 18 months. This requirement does not fully reflect the principles of high reliability, which would expect an organization to continually scan the environment for the identification and reduction of potential risks. We will be trying to help organizations to use proactive risk identification and reduction techniques more regularly in their organizations.

We also want to help organizations rethink their adoption of the elements in our SE Policy. Our definition of SE includes the words "or risk thereof." But events that we ask be reported to the Joint Commission ("reviewable" SEs) are only those that have resulted in serious, permanent harm or death. Each organization is to define for itself the SEs it wants to report internally, but many have included only "reviewable" SEs in their definition. This has resulted in a lot of hospitals not learning from near miss or hazards.

We want to help health care organizations to shift to a broader view of what kinds of events they should investigate and learn from. No one seems to have the final answer yet about how to do this. A consultant to the U.S. Department of Energy has told us that you want to intensively investigate those events, hazards, or incidents that are the most "information rich." Sometimes the most information rich events may be a hazard or a close call, rather than an actual adverse event.

Currently, every SE tends to be analyzed in a silo in which each event is separately evaluated with a RCA. But even if you were to correct every one of an event's identified causes and eliminate them, you have primarily prevented that one particular event from occurring in exactly the same way. Therefore, we are also exploring how an organization can aggregate the results of multiple RCAs so that patterns of causes can be better understood to increase the robustness of interventions.

As to Lean and Six Sigma as RPI tools, when Mark Chassin became President of Joint Commission, he brought with him the experiences from work he had done previously. What he had learned was that people were trying to solve a problem by seeing what others had done to solve the problem. They would then say, "Let's try that here." But often, the borrowed solution was implemented without achieving the same level of success or the sustainability that was experienced by the original organization. In reality, any given problem usually has a number of different causes and these causes are different in different organizations. What was really needed was a solution that was targeted toward the *specific* causes for the problem in the learning hospital.

An example is the Hand Hygiene Project of the Center for Transforming Healthcare, a subsidiary of The Joint Commission. As part of the project, eight voluntary health care organizations first discovered that their beliefs about their hand-hygiene rates were not accurate. They thought they had 80 percent to 90 percent compliance rates; after they used a standardized method to measure their hand-hygiene rates, they discovered that their real rate was 48 percent!

The results of their use of RPI tools for measuring and identifying each hospital's hospital-specific causes were impressive. Causes were different for every organization. Table 3.1 shows that not a single cause was present in all of the hospitals, and no two hospitals had the same pattern of causes.

Our belief is that most hospitals do not have the resources to use all the tools of RPI, such as Lean and Six Sigma methodologies. Therefore, the center has devised an online diagnostic tool and education program that an accredited hospital can use to determine what its own causes are, and then go to the center's database to see what solutions

TABLE 3.1
Hand Hygiene Project: Main Causes of Failure to Clean Hands

MAIN CAUSES OF FAILURE TO CLEAN HANDS (ACROSS ALL PARTICIPATING HOSPITALS)	A	B	C	D	E	F	G	H
Ineffective placement of dispensers or sinks		X		X	X		X	X
Hand hygiene compliance data are not collected or reported accurately or frequently	X	X		X	X			X
Lack of accountability and just-in-time coaching		X	X	X	X		X	X
Safety culture does not stress hand hygiene at all levels			X	X	X	X		X
Ineffective or insufficient education		X	X	X	X		X	
Handsfull	X	X	X	X	X		X	
Wearing gloves interferes with process	X	X	X	X			X	
Perception that hand hygiene is not needed if wearing gloves	X		X	X	X		X	X
Health care workers forget	X	X		X			X	
Distractions	X	X				X	X	

Note that not all of the main causes of failure appear in every hospital. The chart above represents the validation of the root causes across hospitals. This underscores the importance of understanding hospital-specific root causes so that appropriate solutions can be targeted.

From *Joint Commission Center for Transforming Healthcare Storyboard*. ©The Joint Commission, 2010. Reprinted with permission.

are specific to those causes. Of course, it would be desirable for every organization to use RPI tools, but not all will be able to.

Q: What does Joint Commission see as the key barriers to achieving a HRO?

A: There are a number of things. First, the training of health care professionals is much siloed. They are not taught how to work in teams. Also, in current training, the notion that "physicians and nurses should not make mistakes" is ingrained as part of their medical professional identity—there is little recognition that "to err is human." So an error becomes something to be ashamed of and to hide. If hidden, errors cannot be learning opportunities.

One of the characteristics of HROs is they have a "sensitivity to operations." In complex systems, like health care organizations, cause and effect are not linear; little causes can have big effects. Staff in HROs watch for these little changes to effectively respond to them before they turn into large adverse outcomes.

In a high-reliability industry, like nuclear power, little changes are easy to notice in the control room. However, in health care, there are so many unexpected things that constantly occur—for example, the patients' responses to interventions—it is hard to pay attention to all of them. Health care may be more like the flight deck of a naval aircraft carrier that has constant unpredictability.

There is, therefore, still a challenge in figuring out how to implement principles of high reliability in the health care environment of constant change. We are still building the knowledge of how to do this.

Finally, we need to have an atmosphere of trust and just responses if we want people to actually report what is going on. There needs to be a safe or "just" culture—which is not the same as a "blame-free culture." Reckless behavior (as opposed to human error or well-intentioned misjudgments) cannot be tolerated in a culture of safety, in which people must have the trust necessary for transparency and reporting.

Canadian Accreditation

Interview with Wendy Nicklin, President and CEO, Accreditation Canada, July 28, 2010.

Q: Describe the framework and process for developing the cultural assessment (Effective Organization) standards

A: Canada introduced a new accreditation program called Qmentum in 2008

Qmentum standards are developed using a combination of research and expert input from client organizations, Accreditation Canada surveyors, and other stakeholders. Following initial research into the topic including how it is addressed by other accreditation bodies, a proposal is developed that identifies the critical quality and safety issues. An advisory committee, made up of members of the above groups, is then convened to review the draft standards and comment on the relevant issues.

Following review by the advisory committee, a pilot test of the standards is conducted, whereby organizations in the field test the standards and accreditation process. A national consultation, where stakeholders can review the standards document and provide feedback, may also be conducted.

Some of the standards include a required organizational practice (ROP). These particular criteria are mandatory.

Excerpt from the Effective Organization (leadership) standards:

Subsection: STRENGTHENING CULTURE AND VALUES

6.0   The organization's leaders monitor and improve client safety culture on an ongoing basis.

6.1   REQUIRED ORGANIZATIONAL PRACTICE: The organization adopts client safety as a written strategic priority or goal.
Guidelines: There is an important connection between organization excellence and safety. Ensuring safety in the provision and delivery of services is among an organization's primary responsibilities to clients, staff and providers. Accordingly, safety should be a formally written component of the organization's strategic objectives. This may be in the form of the strategic plan, the annual report, or list of organizational goals.

6.2   REQUIRED ORGANIZATIONAL PRACTICE: The organization develops and implements a client safety plan and implements improvements to client safety as required.
Guidelines: Client safety may be improved when organizations consider and develop a plan for addressing safety issues. Safety plans consider the safety issues related to the organization, delivery of services, and needs of clients and families. The safety plan includes a range of topics and approaches for addressing and evaluating safety issues. Safety plans include content such as mentoring staff and service providers, role of leadership (e.g., client safety leadership walkabouts), implementing organization-wide client safety initiations, accessing evidence and best practice, and recognizing staff and service providers for innovations to improve client safety.

6.3   The organization's leaders assign responsibility for implementing and monitoring the client safety plan, and leading client safety improvement activities.
Guidelines: Responsibility for the client safety plan may be assigned to a council, committee, or team whose mandate includes organization-wide client safety; designated staff with responsibility for client safety; or client safety champions whose mandate is to facilitate and improve client safety throughout the organization or within specific work areas.

6.8   ACCREDITATION CANADA REQUIRED INSTRUMENT: The organization monitors its client safety culture by using the Patient Safety Culture Instrument.

Guidelines: The organization's leaders recognize their responsibility for promoting a culture of client safety, for preventing incidents and adverse events, for allocating resources to improve safety, and for fostering a no-blame culture that encourages learning from errors and mistakes. The Patient Safety Culture Instrument is a tool that measures these and other elements to determine organizational commitment to client safety. The organization shares the results of the Patient Safety Culture Instrument with staff and service providers and is able to demonstrate that the results have been used to improve client safety.

Q: How long have the cultural standards been in place?

A: Since a focus on quality improvement is inherent within accreditation, it has always been a component of the Accreditation Canada Program. Fundamentally, our accreditation standards (whether within the leadership or clinical standards) have supported the development and sustainability of a culture focused on quality and safety for many years.

Introduced within the Qmentum program in 2007, for use by organizations beginning in 2008, the Effective Organization (leadership) standards contain many references to organization culture. The specific ROP regarding safety culture was introduced in 2005 within the previous program and subsequently carried over to Qmentum.

Q: From the experience in measuring compliance to the cultural assessment (Effective Organization) standards, what areas have been the most frequent to require improvement?

A: Overall, compliance with standards related to an organization's client safety culture has been quite high. Based on 2009 data, compliance with the criteria (outlined above) relating to client safety culture is between 86 percent and 94 percent.

The Patient Safety Culture Instrument was used by 68 percent of client organizations in 2009 to self-evaluate culture.

Q: Has any research been conducted to show the correlation of culture with patient safety (e.g., measuring number of adverse events with correlation to culture?)

A: Accreditation Canada does not currently collect information about client organizations' adverse or SE occurrences in relation to the patient safety culture of the organization. Qmentum standards, however, recognize the importance of a culture of safety to increasing quality of services, as evidenced by criteria 6.1, 6.2, 6.3, and 6.8, referenced above.

The Effective Organization standards require that organizations report on and monitor the occurrence of adverse events and SEs within their organization, and use the information gathered to make improvements to services.

Given the 3-year cycle of the Accreditation Canada Qmentum Program that was introduced in 2008, by the conclusion of 2010, our database will be such that we can begin to examine correlations between many of the standards and requirements.

Q: What is the scope of the Canadian survey process (how many health care systems are surveyed each year)?

A: Our total client base is approximately 1,200, with more than 3,000 sites included. Approximately 300 to 400 client organizations are surveyed each year in the 3-year cycle. Our client base extends from small community-based organizations to large regional health systems (inclusive of long-term care, quaternary care, home care, and so on). We also survey both public and private organizations.

Q: Are there any standards that address compliance with patient safety goals? If so, what are they?

A: Effective Organization standard 6.0, "The organization's leaders monitor and improve client safety culture on an ongoing basis," speaks specifically to the need to identify patient safety goals and to provide resources and support to achieve those goals. Elements of this standard include creating a client safety plan, assigning responsibility for implementing the plan, carrying out client safety–related prospective analyses, reporting and disclosing adverse and SE occurrences, monitoring the client safety culture of the organization, and providing the governing body with reports on client safety and recommendations for improvements.

Throughout the entire Qmentum program, and as previously noted, there are also ROPs. Compliance with the ROPs is a requirement. In addition to the Effective Organization (leadership) standards, these ROPs are integrated into many different sets of standards as well including governance and the clinical standards. The ROPs address key elements of quality and patient safety within health care organizations. Across the program, there are 35 ROPs, addressing such matters as education and training regarding client safety, medication reconciliation, preventing workplace violence, infection control, and adverse events reporting and disclosure. Our website, www.accreditation.ca, provides details regarding these ROPs.

Q: Please describe Canada's Focus on Patient Safety: ROPs in Qmentum.

A: ROPs are evidence-based practices (EBPs) that mitigate risk and contribute to improving the quality and safety of health services. Accreditation Canada convened a Patient Safety Advisory Committee in 2003 to guide the patient safety–related aspects of the accreditation program. This resulted in an ROP strategy that identified priority areas and integrated the first 21 ROPs into the accreditation program in 2006.

Since 2006, 14 additional ROPs have been introduced, identified with input from health care experts including practitioners, researchers, policy makers, academics, and health service providers. Ongoing ROP development targets high-risk areas in specific health care sectors, whereas existing ROPs are continually refined to increase specificity across the continuum of care and to incorporate emerging evidence from the field.

The ROPs are integrated into the appropriate standards and are organized according to patient safety goal areas. The patient safety goal areas for the ROPs in effect for on-site surveys conducted in 2010 are safety culture, communication, medication use, worklife/ workforce, infection control, and risk assessment. ROPs have a direct impact on an organization's accreditation decision/result. Organizations must meet all the ROP requirements. If they do not, then they must submit evidence to Accreditation Canada within a specified time period outlining how unmet ROPs are being addressed.

The implementation and monitoring of ROPs is one of the many ways that Accreditation Canada plays a central role in ongoing quality improvement and encourages the highest quality care.

Q: Can you provide more information regarding the "worklife" measurements as part of the accreditation requirements?

A: It is widely recognized that the health care environment is one of the most difficult within which to work, because of the physical and emotional demands of the work, the high risk of work-related injury, workload, and work schedules, the increasing acuity of the patients/clients and the high rate of change in the work environment. Accreditation Canada has made an organizational commitment to supporting and enhancing quality worklife in health care. This is reflected in our values statement:

> Within an environment focused on clients and committed to QWL, partnerships and personal growth, our values are excellence, integrity, respect, and innovation.

In 1999, the concept of "worklife" was introduced into the definition of "quality" used by Accreditation Canada, and content regarding worklife was first included in the accreditation standards. In 2003, after further review of the worklife content and results of accreditation surveys that occurred in 2002, Accreditation Canada developed a Worklife Strategy.

The goals of the strategy were as follows:

Provide action plans to improve worklife in organizations

Include worklife content in more standard sections

Develop and provide indicators

Keep worklife outcomes "people focused"

As part of this strategy, a Worklife Advisory Committee was formed that same year to advise Accreditation Canada on future directions regarding worklife. The Committee included 17 experts from the field—researchers, policy advisors, and senior management—who guided the development of the worklife model. The model focuses on the impact on staff, the organization, and patient outcomes of organizational factors, care and service processes, staff characteristics, and patient characteristics.

One of the key steps in this work was to include "Worklife" as one of the eight quality dimensions on which the Qmentum accreditation program standards are based:

1. Population focus: Working with communities to anticipate and meet needs
2. Accessibility: Providing timely and equitable services
3. Safety: Keeping people safe
4. Worklife: Supporting wellness in the work environment
5. Client-centered services: Putting clients and families first
6. Continuity of services: Experiencing coordinated and seamless services

7. Effectiveness: Doing the right thing to achieve the best possible results

8. Efficiency: Making the best use of resources

Standards "tagged" to the worklife quality dimension, or otherwise related to worklife, appear throughout the Qmentum program:

Sustainable Governance Standards

3.0   The governing body defines values for the organization that are used to guide decision making and for determining how services are delivered.

    3.1   The governing body seeks input from staff and service providers to define or update the organization's value statement.

9.0   The governing body works effectively with the CEO, senior management, and clinical leadership to achieve the strategic goals and objectives and improve the organization's performance.

    9.6   The governing body, with the CEO, communicates with staff and the rest of the organization.

16.0   The governing body fosters and supports a culture of safety throughout the organization.

    16.3   The governing body approves policies and initiatives that encourage open communication, blame-free dialogue, and full disclosure about client safety issues, incidents, and potential problems.

Effective Organization (leadership) standards

4.0   The organization's leaders develop and implement the operational plans, infrastructure, and management systems to meet the scope of services and achieve the strategic goals and objectives.

    4.3   When developing the operational plans, the organization's leaders seek input from staff, service providers, volunteers, and other stakeholders, and communicate the plans throughout the organization.

8.0   The organization's leaders promote a positive worklife culture and support worklife balance.

    8.1   The organization has a positive worklife culture as a strategic priority.

8.2   The organization's leaders promote worklife balance.

8.3   The organization has healthy workplace strategies to help staff and service providers manage their health.

8.4   The organization's leaders monitor staff and service providers' fatigue and stress levels, and work to reduce safety issues associated with fatigue and stress.

8.6   The organization has a confidential process for staff, service providers, and volunteers to bring forward complaints, concerns, and grievances.

8.7   The organization's leaders identify and monitor process and outcome measures related to worklife and the working environment.

12.0   The organization invests in its people and in the development of competencies among its senior leaders, staff, service providers, and volunteers.

12.1   The organization's leaders recruit and select staff according to the services the organization provides, organizational goals and objectives, equity, and individual qualifications.

12.2   The organization's leaders implement staff retention strategies for managers, staff, service providers, and volunteers.

12.3   The organization's leaders use a staffing process that is evidence-based and makes appropriate use of individual skills, education, and knowledge.

12.4   The organization's leaders define reporting relationships for staff, service providers, and volunteers.

12.8   The organization's leaders regularly evaluate reporting relationships and managers' span of control.

12.9   The organization's leaders implement policies and procedures to monitor performance.

12.11   The organization's leaders conduct exit interviews with individuals and use this information to improve staffing and retention strategies.

Sector and Service-Based Standards

5.0   The team promotes the well-being and worklife balance of each of its members.

5.1   The organization has defined criteria that are used to assign team members to clients and other responsibilities in a fair and equitable manner.

5.2   Team members have input on work and job design, including the definition of roles and responsibilities, and case assignments, where appropriate.

5.5   The team has a fair and objective process to recognize team members for their contributions.

Accreditation Canada continues to support developments in healthy and quality worklife in health care through its participation in the Quality Worklife Quality Healthcare Collaborative (QWQHC), a coalition of 12 Canadian health care organizations committed to creating healthier workplaces.

Worklife Pulse

The Worklife Pulse survey tool was developed in collaboration with the Ontario Hospital Association (OHA) and builds on the earlier Healthy Hospital Employee Survey (HHES) that was developed by the OHA and Brock University. The goal of the survey tool is to enable organizations to monitor key worklife areas, including measures of QWL determinants and outcomes for individual employee health and the overall organization. Indeed, the Worklife Pulse Survey provides an objective "measure" of how some of the related standards are being met. It helps organizations identify strengths and gaps in their work environments, engage stakeholders in discussions of high priority opportunities for improvement, plan appropriate interventions to improve the QWL, and develop a clearer understanding of how quality worklife influences an organization's capacity to meet its strategic goals.

All staff and physicians within the organization are urged to complete this survey. The survey is composed of 21 items, measuring elements of the work environment, individual QWL, and organizational performance. For most elements, respondents are asked to rate items on a 5-point scale from *strongly disagree* to *strongly agree*, for example:

- I am satisfied with communications in this organization.
- I have enough time to do my job adequately.
- I feel I can trust this organization.
- Working conditions in my area contribute to patient safety.

The Worklife Pulses survey tool became a required component of Accreditation Canada's accreditation program in 2008. Organizations are expected to conduct this survey once in the 3-year accreditation cycle. If the organization's leadership team chooses to administer it annually, that is supported. At the same time, rather than replace an organizations' existing in-depth staff satisfaction survey, the Worklife Pulse survey is intended to be complementary to it.

Australian Accreditation

According to Brian W. Johnston, Chief Executive of the Australian Council on Healthcare Standards (ACHS), August 9, 2010 (B. W. Johnston, Personal Communication, August 9, 2010):

> Healthcare in Australia has had a long and progressive journey to provide excellence in standards—and the Australian Council on Healthcare Standards plays a pivotal role in shaping this continual evolution.

Promoting the concepts of safety, quality and performance in the delivery of health care have been the aim of the Council and its growth as the leading accreditation organization for health care standards in Australia confirms its success in this.

For more than 35 years, the ACHS has played a leading role in promoting quality health care. It has done this through its internationally regarded EQuIP with its basis on standards that are achievable, but stretch performance targets, are evidence-based and reflect industry and community expectations.

It has made an important contribution towards the Australian health industry encouraging it to pursue progressively higher standards of performance.

Whether it is in the public hospital system, in private hospitals, day surgery hospitals or in a range of other health settings, the ACHS accreditation system has assisted in providing a very clear framework for action to make the goals of continual improvement for a range of health care organizations possible.

The ACHS continues to expand its presence on the international health stage. The adoption of the EQuIP program in New Zealand, South-East Asia, the Middle East, India, and beyond indicates the regard in which the ACHS, and the effectiveness of EQuIP, is held.

The ACHS's mission remains to improve the quality and safety of health care.

The following questions and answers regarding the Australian Accreditation System were provided by Ian McManus, communications manager, on behalf of Mr. Brian W. Johnston, Chief Executive of the ACHS, August 9, 2010.

Q: How does the Australian accreditation system measure adverse events?

A: As our indicator sets are specialty specific, adverse events are addressed in a number of indicator sets, including the following:

- Gastrointestinal endoscopy set (eight indicators address adverse events)
- Gynaecology set (seven indicators address adverse events)
- Hospital-wide set (five indicators address adverse events)
- Infection control set (two indicators address adverse events)
- Medication safety set (three indicators address adverse events)
- Mental health inpatient set (nine indicators address adverse events)
- Obstetric set (one indicator addresses adverse events)
- Radiology set (two indicators address adverse events)
- Surgical set (four indicators address adverse events)

The federal government is currently developing a set of national core indicators for hospital inpatients, and these address:

- Hospital standardized mortality ratios
- Death in low-mortality diagnosis–related groups
- In-hospital mortality rates
- Unplanned hospital re-admissions
- Obstetric trauma

All Australian hospitals have policies and procedures addressing adverse events, mostly actual but they are starting to address near misses, however, they rely on self-reporting which has and will always remain an issue.

A major study was conducted in Australia in 1995 addressing the rate of adverse events and is still referenced today in international papers (Wilson et al., 1995).

Q: What is the ACHS?

A: The ACHS is an independent, not-for-profit organization, dedicated to improving the quality and safety of health care in Australia through continual review of performance, assessment and accreditation.

Established in 1974, after many years of pioneering work from a range of health care professionals including members of the Australian Medical Association, medical colleges and the Australian Hospital (now Healthcare) Association, the ACHS has maintained its position as the principal independent authority on the measurement and implementation of quality improvement systems for Australian health care organizations.

The ACHS EQuIP (see Figure 3.1) was launched in 1996 providing health care organizations with an organization-wide framework to deliver a consumer-centered service. The framework includes standards, a self-assessment process, and systematic external peer review.

EQuIP was developed by the ACHS to help health care organizations strive for excellence and was designed to be used by all types of organizations which provide health care. The ACHS assists health care organizations to prepare for ACHS accreditation by guiding them through EQuIP.

The focus of ACHS accreditation programs is to provide a framework for continuous improvement. It is about establishing a structure and processes that allow quality and safety to proliferate.

Over 750 health care organizations representing more than 1,000 individual organizations are members of ACHS quality improvement programs. EQuIP members are from a range of health care organizations such as the following: hospitals, day procedure centers, community health services, specialist care services, rural and remote health services, area/district/network services, and so on.

ACHS Comparative Report Service (Clinical Indicator Program)

The ACHS clinical indicator program is a service offered to health care organizations in Australia and New Zealand. Information from the indicators is the largest source of data gathered on the quality of health care in Australia and New Zealand. It is the only national clinical indicator program which examines data across a full range of medical disciplines.

FIGURE 3.1
The EQuIP cycle.

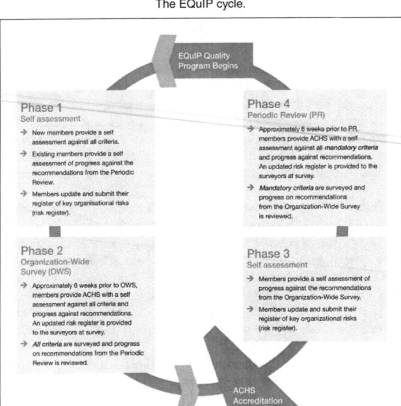

The role of the ACHS Performance and Outcomes Service (POS) is to coordinate the development, collection, collation, analysis, and reporting of the clinical indicators.

The ACHS, through the POS, has considerable information on more than 300 clinical indicators with more than 700 health care organizations participating in the ACHS Comparative Report Service in any 6-month period.

CONCLUSIONS

Patient safety is a global concern. Accreditation programs are increasing in numbers around the world, and each one has variation in standards and their approach to implementing patient safety standards. Canada's measurement of the QWL aims to create an engaged workforce. Australia's EQuIP model has an accreditation cycle of 4 years and measures adverse events through the use of extensive sets of indicators. It is recommended that all health care professionals study global accreditation systems to learn about the variation in methods that drive patient safety and quality using the accreditation process.

REFERENCES

Australian Patient Safety Foundation. (n.d.). *Australian Patient Safety Foundation*. Retrieved from http://www.apsf.net.au/

Baker, G. R., Norton, P. G., Flintoft, V., Blais, R., Brown, A., Cox, J . . . Tamblyn R. (2004). The Canadian Adverse Events Study: The incidence of adverse events among hospital patients in Canada. *Canadian Medical Association*. Retrieved from http://www.cmaj.ca/cgi/content/full/170/11/1678

Canadian Patient Safety Institute. (n.d.). *Building a safer health system*. Retrieved from http://www.patientsafetyinstitute.ca/english/about/Pages/default.aspx

Don't put faith in hospital care, expert warns. (2008, October 28) *The Australian*. Retrieved from http://www.theaustralian.com.au/news/nation/dont-put-faith-in-hospital-care/story-e6frg6nf-1111117879436

Flin, R., Winter, J., Sarac, C., & Raduma, M. (2009). *Human factors in patient safety: Review of topics and tools*. Geneva, Switzerland: WHO.

Gagnon, L. (2004). Medical error affects nearly 25% of Canadians. *Canadian Medical Association Journal*. Retrieved from http://www.cmaj.ca/cgi/content/full/171/2/123-a

IV Team. (2008, August 14). *Medical errors in Japan*. Retrieved from http://www.ivteam.com/medical-errors-in-japan/

Johnston, B.W. (2010). Personal communication papers. Australian Council on Healthcare Standards.

Medical Error Action Group. (2008). *Patient death toll worse than 45 plane crashes per year*. Retrieved from http://www.medicalerroraustralia.com/

National Patient Safety Agency. (2010). *National Patient Safety Agency: About us*. Retrieved from http://www.npsa.nhs.uk/corporate/about-us/

Office of Inspector General. (n.d.). *About the office of Inspector General*. Retrieved from http://oig.hhs.gov/organization.asp

PR Newswire. (2010, November 16). *Report finds medical errors more common & more deadly than previously estimated*. Retrieved from http://www.prnewswire.com/news-releases/report-finds-medical-errors-more-common--more-deadly-than-previously-estimated-108429984.html

Schoen, C., Osborn, R., Huynh, P. T., Doty, M., Zapert, K., & Paugh, J. (2005). *Taking the pulse of health care systems: Experiences of patients with health problems in six countries. The Commonwealth Fund.* Retrieved from http://www.commonwealthfund.org/Publications/In-the-Literature/2005/Nov/Taking-the-Pulse-of-Health-Care-Systems–Experiences-of-Patients-with-Health-Problems-in-Six-Countri.aspx

Shaw, C. D. (2004). *Toolkit for accrediting programs.* Australia: ISQUA.

Soichero, N., Masahiro, K., & Yoshinori, N. (2009). *Healthcare safety committee in Japan: Mandatory accountability reporting system and punishment.* Retrieved from http://journals.lww.com/co-anesthesiology/Fulltext/2009/04000/Healthcare_safety_committee_in_Japan__mandatory.11.aspx

Wilson, R. M., Runciman, W. B, Gibberd, R. W., Harrison, B. T., Newby, L., & Hamilton, J. D. (1995). The quality in Australian Health Care Study. *Medical Journal of Australia*, p. *163*, pp. 458–471.

WHO. (2004). *World Alliance for Patient Safety Forward Programme.* Retrieved from http://www.who.int/patientsafety/en/

WHO. (2006). *Quality of care: A process for making strategic choices in health systems.* Retrieved from http://www.wpro.who.int/health_topics/quality_patient_safety/

WHO. (n.d.-a). *About WHO.* Retrieved from http://www.who.int/about/en/

WHO. (n.d.-b) *Patient safety: Information center.* Retrieved from http://www.who.int/patientsafety/information_centre/en/

Woolcock, N., & Henderson, M. (2004, August 13). Blundering hospitals kill 40,000 a year: One in ten treated by NHS falls victim to errors, officials admit. *The Sunday Times.* Retrieved from http://www.timesonline.co.uk/tol/news/uk/article468980.ece

4

Universal "New" Language of Patient Safety as Part of the Accreditation Process: Review of Terms

*A*ccording to published reports such as those in Consumers Union (2009), we know that health care continues to be "unsafe." As many as 100,000 preventable deaths occur per year as the result of medical harm. This number translates into over 1 million preventable deaths and billions of dollars wasted over the past 10 years.

However, the capacity for the health care system to continually learn from honest mistakes depends on the effectiveness of the reporting systems.

Edwards Deming believed that blaming individuals does little to correct the variation within the system that produced the results observed. He promoted constant learning and continual improvement of processes (Deming, 1982).

The accreditation process of the Joint Commission requires health care providers to apply concepts of patient safety, which includes identifying and learning from medical mistakes and harm. For health care organizations to effectively apply concepts of patient safety, a new language must be learned.

The following are some of the key critical terms one needs to know when applying patient safety concepts:

Error: According to Reason (1990), error is caused by a failure to plan correctly or execute a correct plan. When mistakes involve a failure to plan, it means that either a mistake has been made, or the wrong plan has been implemented, or the outcome is not as intended. Mistakes involve conscious reasoning and planning, typically through knowledge deficits, or a failure to correctly process information or to correctly apply a rule. In effect, mistakes involve faulty problem solving of some kind. Preventive methods for errors involving mistakes in planning should always focus on increased supervision, training, and remedial education (when dealing with a knowledge deficit).

For example, a new nurse graduate is assigned to care for a postoperative patient. The patient's pulse continues to elevate and the patient feels anxious. The nurse thinks the patient is just nervous. The patient's blood pressure suddenly drops and the patient suffers a cardiac arrest and ends up in the intensive care unit because the nurse failed to process the information correctly owing to her knowledge deficit.

Slips and lapses: Slips and lapses can cause poor outcomes when the correct plan is implemented incorrectly. Slips and lapses are errors involving skill-based behaviors. These are the kinds of behaviors exhibited so frequently that the person goes on "autopilot" when performing them (Human Factors MD, 2010).

Slips and lapses may be due to a lack of concentration caused by distraction, stress, fatigue, or competing sensory inputs. For example, a nurse is preparing medications. She gets distracted by an interruption and places the wrong medication in a medicine cup. She then administers the wrong medication to a patient.

Another example of a slip and lapse is when a surgeon is tired because he has worked excessive hours the past week. He accidentally nicks a vessel when performing a surgery in which he has extensive experience. Preventive methods for this type of error include reducing work hours to prevent fatigue, designing equipment and devices in a manner that reduces variation, eliminating distractions when work is performed, and other systems redesign efforts (AHRQ, n.d.).

Adverse event: An adverse event is an injury caused by medical care (AHRQ, n.d.). Adverse events are not caused by the patient's underlying medical condition. Many errors do not result in adverse events and, as a result, a proportion of medical errors are not even detected for learning opportunities.

The IHI has a tool for measuring adverse events and is free for download at www.ihi.org/IHI/Results/WhitePapers/IHIGlobalTrigger ToolWhitePaper.htmt.

Errors of commission and omission: An error of commission involves a wrong action. An error of omission involves no action when action was needed (Joint Commission, 2006). In other words, an error of commission is doing the wrong thing and an error of omission is failing to act to do the right thing.

For example, a nurse administering 10 times the normal dosage of a medication to a patient, which results in a patient's death, is an error of commission. A nurse forgetting to administer a stat antibiotic to a patient who has early sepsis, which results in the patient requiring respiratory support in intensive care, is an error of omission.

Both errors of commission and omission may or may not result in patient harm depending on the effect of the error or timely intervention, for example, a patient receiving the wrong medication but not experiencing any ill effects because of this error. This may be due to chance and the patient's unique response to the medication.

An example of timely intervention is when a nurse administers the wrong medication and quickly realizes her wrong actions, notifies the physician, and administers a medication that counteracts the potential ill effects of the first medication administered.

Sentinel Event: "An unexpected occurrence involving death or serious physical or psychological injury, or the risk thereof" (Joint Commission, n.d.).

SEs involve serious injuries with loss of limb or function. Joint Commission maintains an online database for SEs reported and updates this database periodically. SEs require RCA with the aim of reducing and/or eliminating the reoccurrence in the future by systems redesign and learning.

Overuse: Wrong actions create circumstances where the potential for harm exceeds the known benefits or there is minimal evidence that demonstrates medical justification, for example, when physicians order antibiotics for the common cold; this overuse can increase antibiotic resistance. Another example is the use of unnecessary diagnostic tests, such as MRIs, when the results will not change the selection of a treatment by the physician (Robert Wood Johnson Foundation, n.d.).

Underuse: The omitted action (failure to act) may prevent a favorable outcome for the patient. For example, the physician does not provide screening for hypertension or, flu shots are not accessible to underserved populations (Robert Wood Johnson Foundation, n.d.).

Misuse: The action selected is appropriate but a preventable complication occurs and the patient does not receive the full benefit of what was intended. This is another way of describing medical errors. For example, a patient has a known allergy to an antibiotic and the physician accidentally orders it anyway; the patient experiences an allergic reaction to the antibiotic and develops a rash (Robert Wood Johnson Foundation, n.d.).

Root cause analysis: Joint Commission requires RCA for SEs that occur in health care systems. The process of RCA requires probing to start at the interface between the health care worker (referred to as the "sharp end") and to continue until this process exposes systems issues (at the "blunt end"). These systems issues, when corrected, may reduce and/or eliminate the risk of reoccurrence. RCA focuses on systems issues and not on individual performance issues (Joint Commission, 2006).

When a credible and thorough RCA is performed, the causal reasons for the SE are identified. So what is a credible and thorough RCA? To be thorough means that the RCA process has covered all the potential areas that may have contributed to the SE. These include the following:

- Determining the human factors along with other factors that are most directly associated with the SE along with the processes and systems that are also related to the SE.
- Requiring a series of "why?" questions to analyze the underlying systems and processes to determine where systems redesign efforts may reduce the risk of reoccurrence.
- Requiring that all areas in the Joint Commission matrix be covered to ensure that all potential areas appropriate to the specific type of event are considered and investigated. The matrix matches categories of SEs to the appropriate areas for further investigation. For example, wrong site surgery would require the following areas for investigation: physical assessment process, patient identification process, staffing levels, orientation and training of staff, competency assessment/credentialing of staff, communication with patient/family, availability of information, and physical environment.
- Identifying the risk points and their linkage to the SE.

This is to determine areas for potential improvement in processes or systems that when implemented are likely to reduce the risk of reoccurrence in the future, or a determination that no such improvement opportunity exists.

To be credible, Joint Commission requires the following:

- Leadership involvement as well as involvement of the staff most closely involved in the process and systems under review.
- Involvement of staff most directly involved in the process and systems is also essential. The team cannot track and compare what happened with what should have happened without involvement of the staff most knowledgeable about the process and systems being investigated.
- The RCA must not leave any obvious question unanswered and must not contradict itself. It must also provide reasonable explanations for all findings, including those that are not applicable or not a current problem.
- The RCA must include a review and consideration of any relevant literature (Joint Commission, n.d.).

For further information regarding RCA for SEs, go to www.joint commission.org and type in the search area: "Sentinel Event policy."

Failure mode and effect analysis (FMEA): Joint Commission requires health care organizations to perform a proactive risk assessment at least every 18 months, and FMEA is one method for accomplishing this task. The goal in FMEA is to prevent adverse events from occurring. Basically, performing FMEA requires that the team have a clear understanding of the steps of the process and map out what might occur (potential failures in each step) and what the effect would potentially be if these steps failed (ASHRM, 2002).

Just culture: Joint Commission (2009) refers to a culture of safety and quality within the leadership chapter. Part of a culture of safety and quality pertains to maintaining a just culture. A just culture means that staff are not punished for making honest mistakes and that "reckless" behavior is handled via administrative channels. Marx (2001) described a method for analysis and decision making by leadership to determine whether disciplinary action is warranted depending on the nature of the person's actions and whether those actions were judged to be reckless.

A just culture is the balance between accountability for the individual and the contributing systems issues. It is not an easy task to accomplish, and health care organizations demonstrate wide variation in their quality and patient safety cultures.

A just culture is one where staff speak up and disclose errors, including their own, although maintaining professional accountability. A just culture is also not tolerant of reckless behavior that involves acting in conscious disregard of clear risks to patients or when gross misconduct occurs.

Negligence: Negligence is when the mistake involves a failure to exercise expected care, and the health care provider should have been aware of substantial risk to the patient when the actions were taken. Legally, the term means to do something that a reasonably prudent person would not do, or the failure to do something that a reasonably prudent person would do under like conditions (Lectric Law Library, n.d.).

Recklessness: Recklessness is when there is a conscious disregard of substantial and unjustifiable risk to the patient and the health care provider does it anyway. Marx described it as "where someone chooses to put others in harm's way" (AHRQ, 2007).

Recklessness is not tolerated within a just culture. If a surgeon knows that he has not previously used a new piece of equipment and uses it in surgery anyway without receiving vendor training and obtainment of competency, this is reckless behavior.

Intentional rule violation: An intentional rule violation occurs when the health care provider knows the rule or procedure but does not follow it. For example, hospital staff know that they are supposed to wash their hands before patient contact, but some do not comply. Marx describes this as "at risk behavior" (AHRQ, 2007).

Sharp end: Sharp end refers to the interface of the health care systems in direct contact with patients: the health care provider operating the equipment, administering treatments and medications, and so forth. When an error occurs at the sharp end, the term "active errors" is used (AHRQ, n.d.).

Blunt end: Blunt end refers to the systems issues (frequently longstanding) that influence patient outcomes. When an error occurs at the blunt end, the term "latent errors" is used (AHRQ, n.d.).

Staffing, competencies, type of equipment chosen for use, communication patterns, and so forth are all examples of issues that are found at the blunt end of the systems. The blunt end surfaces with RCA questioning, drills down from the sharp end, and continues on to the blunt end in the search for contributing causes to the adverse event.

Near miss: Near miss means that the fact that the event did not cause patient harm was only by chance or timely intervention (AHRQ, n.d.). Near miss events are reported within health care organizations and matched with potential severity scores that rank potential future harm if the event occurs again. The use of near miss events enhances organizational learning and proactively reduces risk to patients.

Safety: Safety refers to being free from harm or risk of harm (usually as a result of mitigation or preventive efforts). The IOM describes safety as the prevention of harm to patients. The harm can occur through commission or omission (Institute of Medicine, 2003).

One of the more extensive vocabularies for patient safety is available at www.psnet.ahrq.gov/glossary.aspx.

CONCLUSIONS

A review and understanding of basic patient safety terms help in applying patient safety concepts as part of the accreditation process. All health care organizations must develop a culture in which staff are not afraid to report their mistakes; otherwise, staff will underreport adverse events and the system will lose its opportunity to learn from the error and correct the underlying conditions that led to the adverse event in the first place. RCA is a tool that assists the health care organization to focus on processes and not people, for the correction of underlying systems issues that, when implemented, reduce future risk to patients.

REFERENCES

Agency for Healthcare Research and Quality. (2007, October). *Perspectives on safety: In conversation with David Marx, JD.* Retrieved January 11, 2011, from http://www.webmm.ahrq.gov/perspective.aspx?perspective ID=49

Agency for Healthcare Research and Quality. (n.d.). *Patient safety network: Glossary.* Retrieved May 6, 2010, from http://www.psnet.ahrq.gov/glossary .aspx

American Society for Healthcare Risk Management. (2002). *Strategies and tips for maximizing failure mode effect analysis in your organization.* Retrieved May 10, 2010, from http://www.hospitalconnect.com/hospitalconnect_app/search/ ashrm_results.jsp?client=ASHRM_FRONTEND&proxystylesheet=ASHRM_ FRONTEND&output=xml_no_dtd&filter=0&oe=ISO-8859-1&q=white+ papers&site=ASHRM&submit=Go

Consumers Union. (2009). *To err is human—to delay is deadly: Ten years later, a million lives lost, billions of dollars wasted.* Retrieved January 2, 2011, from http:// www.safepatientproject.org/safepatientproject.org/pdf/safepatientproject .org-ToDelayIsDeadly.pdf

Deming, W. E. (1982). *Out of crisis.* Cambridge, MA: Massachusetts Institute of Technology.

Human Factors MD. (2010). *The psychology of error.* Retrieved January 11, 2011, from http://www.humanfactorsmd.com/hfandmedicine_reducerror_nature.html

Institute of Medicine. (2003). *Patient safety: Achieving a new standard.* Washington, DC: National Academy Press.

Joint Commission. (2006). *Sentinel event glossary of terms.* Retrieved May 6, 2010, from http://www.jointcommission.org/sentinelevents/se_glossary.htm

Joint Commission. (2006). *Sentinel event glossary of terms.* Retrieved May 10, 2010, from http://www.jointcommission.org/SentinelEvents/se_glossary.htm

Joint Commission. (2009). *Hospital accreditation standards.* Oakbrook Terrace, IL: Joint Commission Resources.

Joint Commission. (n.d.). *Joint commission: Sentinel events.* Retrieved May 6, 2010, from http://www.jointcommission.org/facts_about_the_sentinel_event_policy/

Lectric Law Library. (n.d.). *Negligence.* Retrieved January 16, 2011, from http://www.lectlaw.com/def2/n010.htm

Marx, D. (2001). *Patient safety and "just culture": Primer for health care executives.* Retrieved May 10, 2010, from http://www.mers-tm.org/support/Marx_Primer.pdf

Reason, J. (1990). *Human error.* New York, NY: Cambridge University Press.

Robert Wood Johnson Foundation. (n.d.). *The state of healthcare quality in America.* Retrieved January 2, 2011, from http://files/research/currentstateofquality.pdf

II

Why a Model Is Needed When Developing and Implementing Patient Safety and Accreditation Initiatives

5

Current Challenges in Health Care

EXTERNAL ENVIRONMENT

According to the American College of Health Care Executives' *Top Issues Confronting Hospitals: 2010*, financial challenges continue to top the list of issues that are of concern to CEOs, with Medicare and Medicaid reimbursement being of special concern.

In 1983, Medicare's prospective payment system of cost reimbursement was introduced, which implemented fixed rates in an effort to create incentives for hospitals to control costs (Mayes & Berenson, 2006). Prior to that, physicians received fee-for-service payment. This type of payment was individualized for each patient according to his or her need with a built-in incentive for the physician to overuse the care provided to patients for profit.

Managed care was developed in the United States as a response to increasing health care costs. Managed care creates responsibility for a defined population with a financial incentive in reducing costs by implementing controls that modify the actions of physicians (Eddy, 1997). This shifting landscape of health care with emphasis on cost savings has demanded that staff work with greater efficiencies while caring for sicker and sicker populations.

COMPLEXITY

The end of World War II started the growth of the medical community and the proliferation of increased specialization (Fillmore, n.d.). Nursing specialization has been patterned after physician specialization in various health care settings. Other health care professionals have also been added with the use of new technologies.

It is not uncommon for a patient who enters a hospital to encounter numerous specialties and varied categories of health care professionals as he or she travels through different levels of care during his or her hospital stay. Every encounter by a health care provider and every transfer the patient experiences through the health care system increases the risk of medical error. The potential for medical error is embedded in the system design.

Increasing use of new technologies, specialization, and new roles creates unique challenges in providing safe care. Health care is becoming increasingly complex and mirrors the growing complexity of the regulatory and external environment. This complexity requires a systems approach to better understand the reasons why breakdowns occur and allow us to move from a blame-and-shame culture to learning, or relearning, and how to identify and correct the vulnerabilities and failures in health care. As a result, we now have Complexity Science, which seeks to clarify how best to use living systems that are nonlinear in nature and that respond and adapt to dynamic, changing environments (Center for the Study of Healthcare Management, 2003).

ETHICS

Lucian Leape stated in 2005 that, of the many challenges to implementing a safer practice environment, the ethical challenges are "among the most profound."

As he put it: "The ethical imperative involves doing all we can realistically to prevent errors and injuries to patients, respond appropriately to adverse events and to seek new ways to prevent reoccurrence. This care requires honesty, openness, and dialogue to ensure that health care professionals are safe and competent."

It is difficult to have honest, open dialogue when positions are stratified in a manner that creates a high degree of differentiation in authority and status. For example, a comparison of the administrative staff with the line staff, or of the physician group with the nursing group, shows a high degree of differentiation in authority and status both within their groups and external to their groups. Added to that are the silos of management structures that tend to produce isolated views pertaining to each group's own departmental view instead of the "big picture" process view.

All providers of health care have the legal and moral obligation to always act in their patients' best interests. This includes full disclosure with alternative options when treatment is offered as well as when outcomes are not as desired.

According to Egan (2004), the common ground of patient safety, ethics, and health care is the emphasis that all three place on improving outcomes.

Accreditation in health care places emphasis on achieving desired outcomes by requiring performance measures to promote quality improvement. According to Chassin, Loeb, Schmaltz, and Wachter (2010), there are four criteria for accountability measures. They should:

1. Be evidence-based.
2. Accurately capture whether the evidence-based care was delivered.
3. Be proximate to the desired outcome with few intervening processes.
4. Ideally have no unintended adverse consequences.

Out of 28 measures that were evaluated according to the four criteria, there were 22 measures that met all the accountability criteria. It is hoped that the use of the criteria as a framework for consensus across the various drivers of performance measures will assist in eliminating measures that do not meet the accountability criteria thereby producing meaningful measurements that will help to save thousands of lives.

STAFFING

Joint Commission (2010) requires that all information from the results of RCA's be reported annually to the hospital's governance. The report includes all actions taken to improve safety, both in response to the event, and to prevent similar events from occurring in the future.

This requirement means that when nurse staffing and/or competency were identified as contributing factors to the adverse event, appropriate actions by the leadership are required. Also, on an annual basis, the leadership is required to review all analyses and actions taken to resolve any staffing problems that have surfaced during the year as the result of RCA results.

NURSE STAFFING

Nurse staffing is a major ethical issue within our health care system. Here, nurse executives must balance expectations for cost constraints, as mandated by boards of directors, and the responsibility to maintain safe, evidence-based nurse-to-staff ratios.

Certainly, nursing salaries make up a big chunk of the operational costs. And as we know, in times of fiscal restraint, salaries are a target for downsizing, restructuring, and reengineering to reduce costs.

High turnover of nursing staff impacts patient safety as well. Nurses are in a learning curve during and after their orientation period. Nurses must learn new procedures and also learn the system's policies for effective communication and actions. For example, the nurse must know how to notify a physician and what to do when the physician does not call back within a reasonable time frame.

In response to the nurse staffing crisis, the Joint Commission published a white paper in 2002 offering the following recommendations: create organizational cultures of retention, bolster the nursing educational infrastructure, and establish financial incentives for investing in nursing to reward effective staffing (Joint Commission, 2002).

The work environment influences nursing satisfaction. Nurses who are dissatisfied search for other job opportunities that better meet their work expectations. High turnovers of nursing staff affect the quality and safety of patient care.

In an extensive job satisfaction survey of 76,000 nurses on elements of job satisfaction reported through the American Nurses Association's (ANA) National Database of Nursing Quality Indicators (NDNQI), registered nurses as a group reported the lowest satisfaction with decision making, tasks, and pay (BNET, 2005).

The AHRQ in 2007 performed a meta-analysis on 96 observational reports to examine the relationship between nurse staffing and outcomes. The results suggested that an increase in registered nurse-to-patient ratios was associated with reduced hospital-related deaths, failure to rescue, and other nurse-sensitive outcomes such as reduced length of stays. Of interest was that the relative risk reduction for every additional full-time equivalent registered nurse, there was a 9 percent risk reduction in hospital-related mortality in intensive care units and a 16 percent reduction of mortality in surgical patients (AHRQ, 2007).

This meta-analysis confirmed previous studies that concluded that increased nurse staffing is associated with better care outcomes. However, this association has not been shown to reflect a causal relationship because hospitals may implement other actions that also improve nursing quality.

Nurse executives continue to struggle within cost containment environments and are forced to make staffing decisions on a daily basis that impact patient safety.

Extended work shifts and mandatory overtime are still being used to cover staffing shortages and provide patient care. The ANA (2010) reported the following results from a survey of approximately 220,000 registered nurses from 13,000 nursing units in over 550 hospitals, with a response rate of 70 percent: 54 percent of nurses in adult medical nursing units and emergency rooms reported that they did not have adequate time with patients, and 43 percent of registered nurses were working extra hours due to shortages in nurse staffing or increased workload. The ANA further reinforced its view that mandated, fixed nursing-to-patient ratios do not allow the flexibility to accommodate changes in technology, competency level of the nurse staffing level and type of support services, or changes in patient needs.

Rogers, Wei-Ting Hwang, Scott, Aiken, and Dinges (2004) reported that the risks of making an error were significantly increased when work shifts were longer than 12 hours, when nurses worked overtime, or when nurses worked in excess of 40 hours per week.

Recognizing that nursing's contribution to care within a health care organization is viewed as an expense, Walton in 2007 described an alternative that proposed reimbursing nursing care based on the intensity level of the care provided instead of bundling it up with fixed costs for room and board per patient.

STAFFING CASE STUDY

The CEO wants to cut nursing salary costs by 10 percent to meet the new budgetary requirements. He has given the nurse executive his mandate. Currently, the nurse executive maintains nurse staffing by the use of float personnel and overtime.

The nurse executive meets with her nursing management team and issues a notice to the nurse managers that no new positions will be filled and that fixed nurse-to-patient ratios will be implemented on the units to avoid use of overtime.

In this all too common example, the nurse executive does not use a systems approach to implement the CEO's mandate. In not using a systems approach, the nurse executive does not take into full account the impact of nurse staffing on patients. Use of a systems approach would have guided the nurse executive to a framework that included gathering appropriate information from risk and utilization management, patient safety, nurses delivering care, the medical group, support areas, and patient satisfaction. The skill mix of the various areas would be examined as well as various nursing care delivery models. The nurse executive would also review all support services to seek opportunities for providing better support to nursing staff on the nursing units. For example, courier service to the laboratory and pharmacy could be provided every 15 to 30 minutes, depending on the acuity of the nursing unit. In effect, all departments would seek ways, by working together, to increase efficiencies by streamlining processes. The change process itself would be monitored, along with each change made, to determine how patient care changed with regular feedback to leadership.

CONCLUSIONS

Health care is increasingly complex and requires a systems approach to problem solving. Processes are not contained within one department but rather cross through many departments to achieve patient outcomes. The health care leadership has an ethical imperative to develop a safer environment in which patient care is provided. This is a challenging task in the midst of competing demands of continued cost reductions and the current organizational architectures that helped to create silos of management structures.

One of the most challenging issues facing health care is the provision of safe and effective nurse staffing. Nursing is the largest piece of the budget pie for salary expense. Cutting nurse staffing has the potential to create unsafe working conditions and increase the risk of the occurrence of adverse events. Staffing requires an evidence-based, ethical, and systems framework when strategic planning is done, and the lack of a systems approach negatively affects the quality of nursing.

REFERENCES

American College of Health Care Executives. (2010). *Research. Top issues confronting hospitals: 2010*. Retrieved January 10, 2011, from http://www.ache.org/pubs/research/ceoissues.cfm

Agency for Healthcare Research and Quality. (2007). *Nurse staffing and quality of patient care*. Evidence report/Technology Assessment No.151 PB No. 07-E005.

American Nurses Association. (2010). *Nursing staffi ng plans and ratios*. Retrieved January 11, 2011, from http://www.nursingworld.org/main menucategories/ANAPoliticalPower/State/StateLegislativeAgenda/StaffingPlansandRatios_1.aspx

BNET. (2005). ANA RN job satisfaction survey of 76,000 nurses probes elements of job satisfaction. Retrieved May 15, 2010, from http://findarticles.com/p/articles/mi_qa3902/is_200506/ai_n13643828/

Center for the Study of Healthcare Management. (2003). *Applying complexity science to health and healthcare*. (Publication 3 Series) Carlson School of Management: University of Minnesota. Retrieved January 11, 2011, from http://www.csom.umn.edu/Assets/11261.pdf

Chassin, M. R., Loeb, J. M., Schmaltz, S. P., & Wachter, R. M. (2010). Accountability measures—using measurement to promote quality improvement. *The New England Journal of Medicine*. Retrieved January 12, 2011, from http://www.nejm.org/doi/full/10.1056/NEJMsb1002320

Eddy, D. M. (1997). Balancing costs and quality in fee-for-service versus managed care. *Health Affairs, 16*(3), 162–173.

Egan, E. A. (2004). The role of ethics and ethics services in patient safety. In B. J. Youngberg & M. J. Hatlie (Eds.), *Patient safety handbook*. Sudbury, MA: Jones and Bartlett.

Fillmore, R. (n.d.). *The evolution of the US Healthcare system*. Retrieved January 10, 2011, from http://www.sciencescribe.net/articles/The_Evolution_of_the_U.S._Healthcare_System.pdf

Joint Commission. (2002). *Health care at the crossroads: Strategies for addressing the evolving nursing crisis.* Retrieved May 16, 2010, from http://www.jointcommission.org/assets/1/18/health_care_at_the_crossroads.pdf

Joint Commission (2010). Comprehensive Accreditation Manual for Hospitals. Joint Commission on Accreditation of Healthcare Organizations.

Leape, L. L. (2005). Ethical issues in patient safety. *Thoracic Surgical Clinic, 15*(4), 493–501.

Mayes, R., & Berenson, R. A. (2006). *Medicare prospective payment and the shaping of U.S. healthcare.* Baltimore, MD: Johns Hopkins University Press.

Rogers, A., Hwang, W., Scott, R. D., Aiken, L., & Dinges, D. (2004). The working hours of hospital staff nurses and patient safety. *Health Affairs, 23*(4), 202–212.

Walton, J. M. (2007). *Mandatory hospital nurse to patient staffing ratios: Time to take a different approach.* Retrieved May 16, 2010, from http://www.nursingworld.org/MainMenuCategories/ANAMarketplace/ANAPeriodicals/OJIN/TableofContents/Volume122007/No3Sept07/MandatoryNursetoPatientRatios.aspx

6

The Reliability Factor and Why Adverse Events Still Happen in Accredited Health Care Organizations

Why do adverse events still occur in accredited hospitals? The Joint Commission has standards related to patient safety linked with leadership standards. Is that enough? Obviously not.

Actually, accreditation provides only a minimal foundation for patient safety efforts. This foundation needs to be slowly raised so that patient safety is the priority and no patient is ever harmed when under a provider's care.

RELIABILITY CONCEPTS

The public is beginning to understand that health care is not reliable. As consumer knowledge increases, so will demands to increase reliability in health care. Preventable harm is just that—preventable. The aim for reliability is perfection on a consistent basis: "to do no harm— all of the time." This means zero failures. According to Nolan, Resar, Haraden, and Griffin (2004), reliability is measured as "number of actions that achieve the intended result ÷ total number of actions taken." Aviation passenger safety for reliability is measured at 10^{-6}. This means that there is only one defect per million attempts. Why cannot health care be this safe, and why should not the public demand it?

Nolan et al. (2004) described a three-tiered strategy for designing systems for reliability. The processes and procedures in place are intended to prevent failure, identify and mitigate failure when it does occur before harm is caused or mitigate the harm caused by failures when they are not detected and intercepted, and to redesign the process based on the critical failures that are identified.

The first level is prevention. Prevention processes involve the use of tools such as standardization (e.g., ordering the same type of equipment, using standardized physician order sets, or protocols), checklists that serve as memory aids, feedback methods for compliance, and continued training. Processes aimed at prevention typically result in a 10^{-1} system, which means the system produces 90 percent compliance, or 1 defect per 10 attempts. When compliance audits are performed, 90 percent compliance may be an organizational target, but successfully meeting the target does not help the 1 out of 10 patients who did not receive the desired care.

The second level involves identification and mitigation. Once 10^{-1} strategies are in place, the second tier can be designed to focus on identifying those events that occur when the standardized method is not sufficient.

Error proofing occurs at this level, which decreases the need for persons to seek work-around solutions. Human factor engineering tools and concepts are used to attain this level of reliability.

The third level involves redesign that is based on the critical failures identified to attain 10^{-3} reliability, which represents 1 defect per 1,000 attempts.

This redesign effort uses failure modes and effects analysis (FMEA) as a method to identify, analyze, and provide solutions for the weaknesses in the processes that are either leading to or have the potential to lead to failure. Risk priority numbers (RPNs) are used to assess risk—the lower the number, the less the risk.

The RPNs decrease dramatically after systematic FMEAs are performed. The IHI provides detailed step-by-step instructions at www.ihi.org/ihi/workspace/tools/fmea on how to conduct an FMEA. Just search FMEA and numerous resources are available.

Six Sigma is a RPI method utilizing statistical analysis that reduces process variation and defects. It was developed to improve the manufacturing processes at Motorola; however, the concepts are used to improve any process. Six Sigma statistically means that there is a failure rate of only 3.4 parts per million, or 99.9997 percent reliability.

HealthEast Care System in St. Paul, Minnesota, was cited by IHI as an example of an organization employing Six Sigma in health care. Wilson et al. (2005) initiated a Six Sigma project with 3M Health Care on a 20-bed medical/surgical intensive care and improved hand hygiene practice compliance from 36 to 70 percent ($p < 0.001$) with a corresponding statistically significant increase in the volume of hand sanitizer used. The complete report for this project is available at www.ihi.org/IHI/Topics/Patient Safety/SafetyGeneral/ImprovementStories/ImprovingHandHygiene PracticewithSixSigma.htm

HEALTH CARE IS NOT RELIABLE

According to Nolan et al. (2004), health care processes function at a level of 10^{-1} (1 defect per 10 attempts). They studied a range of international studies pertaining to adverse events that occur in hospitals that demonstrated an agreement around an error rate of 10 percent with only a plus- or minus-^{2} variation. At the other end are the nuclear power plants having a reliability of 10^{-6} (one defect per million attempts), which makes them HROs.

In the book *Normal Accidents: Living with High Risk Technologies*, Perrow (1984) concluded that in highly complex organizations where processes are tightly coupled, it is not a question of *if* catastrophic accidents will happen but *when* they will happen. Perrow coined the phrase "normal accidents." In the book, he discusses the accident at Three Mile Island in 1979.

One factor in risk assessment is tight coupling, which is when the subcomponents of the system have prompt and major impacts on each other. This means that there are multiple, critical dependencies that create effects that are difficult to anticipate. An example of this in health care is during surgery when a patient's quickly deteriorating condition warrants immediate actions by numerous members of the team to respond simultaneously.

According to Roberts (n.d.), aviation was the first area to develop HRO-like principles after a deadly airplane crash in Portland in 1978. Most of the airline industry companies implemented some form of CRM, which teaches flight attendants, pilots, and other aviation workers how to communicate effectively with each other. Also, CRM reduces status differentials within the flight crew, allowing the person with the expertise to be the decision maker regardless of rank or position.

CRM training in health care grew from health care's recognition that the need for teamwork training might assist with creating a safer work environment by focusing on communication and situational awareness among team members, particularly in areas such as operating rooms and critical care areas (Agency for Healthcare Research and Quality [AHRQ], n.d.).

According to AHRQ (2004), high-reliability organizing concepts involve five characteristics that need to guide the thinking process of people who work in an HRO. They are as follows:

1. *Sensitivity to operations:* HROs know that manuals and policies constantly change and are keenly aware of the complexity of the systems in which they work. The maintenance of situational awareness is important for staff at all levels because this is the only way that detection of actual or potential errors can be quickly identified and fixed before the consequences become much larger. There is a quick response to small changes in which staff recognizes and reacts quickly.

2. *Reluctance to simplify:* HROs do not accept simplistic answers for challenges that confront them. They recognize that their work is complex and that they cannot identify all of the ways in which their systems could fail in the future. There is cultivation for multiple perspectives.

3. *Preoccupation with failure:* HROs are focused on preventing failures rather than reacting to them. They are proactive and constantly entertain "what if?" scenarios. Near misses are viewed as learning opportunities to prevent future failure from occurring. When small events go wrong, this is viewed as the warning before a major catastrophic event occurs.

4. *Deference to expertise:* HROs create and maintain a culture in which team members and organizational leaders defer to the person who possesses the most knowledge of the issue they are confronting. Staff feel comfortable with speaking up to share concerns with others. This means that there is a flexible hierarchy in which authority lines shift to the person with the knowledge to carry out the task, not necessarily the person who is senior ranking.

5. *Resilience:* Leaders and staff pay close attention to their ability to quickly contain errors and innovate when difficulties occur. The system can function even when there are problems. Staff are continuously trained in how to respond when things go wrong and can perform quick situational assessments.

HEALTH CARE IS AN HRO OR *NOT*?

Health care has a very long way to go to be an HRO. Medical mistakes also occur with diagnoses and these diagnostic errors can lead to tragic consequences.

Just how reliable are the physicians' diagnoses?

An article in the March 11, 2009, issue of the *Journal of the American Medical Association* contained Dr. Newman-Toker and Dr. Pronovost's commentary that misdiagnosis accounts for an estimated 40,000 to 80,000 hospital deaths per year and that tort claims for diagnostic errors—defined as diagnoses that are missed, wrong, or delayed— are actually almost twice as common as claims for errors involving medications and involve high payouts.

Equally disturbing are clear indications of unreliable diagnostic testing even before the patient enters the hospital. Hickner et al. (2007) reported about the types and outcomes of the testing process errors that occur in primary care settings. The study involved 243 clinicians and office staff of 8 family medicine offices with the main outcome measures being distribution of error types, associations with potential predictors, predictors of harm, and consequences of the errors.

There were 590 event reports with 966 testing process errors. Errors occurred in ordering tests (12.9 percent), implementing tests (7.9 percent), reporting the test results to clinicians (24.6 percent), clinicians responding to results (6.6 percent), notifying the patient of the results (6.8 percent), general administration (17.6 percent), communication (5.7 percent), and other categories (7.8 percent). Charting or filing errors were found to be 14.5 percent.

Significant results ($p < 0.05$) also were present for error types and type of reporter (clinician or staff), number of labs used by the practice, absence of a follow-up system, and the patients' race/ethnicity.

Adverse clinical outcomes included time lost and financial consequences (22 percent), delays in care (24 percent), pain and suffering (11 percent), and adverse clinical consequences (2 percent). In 54 percent of the events, patients were unharmed, 18 percent resulted in some harm, and for 28 percent the harm was unknown.

The authors used multilevel regression analysis and reported that adverse consequences of harm were more common in events that were clinician reported, for patients who were of age 45 to 64 and involved test implementation errors. Of note was that minority patients were more likely than white, non-Hispanic patients to suffer adverse consequences or harm.

INJURY UNDERREPORTING

Even the health care environment is not safe for new medical school graduates enrolled in surgical residencies; this group may be at high risk for hepatitis and HIV infections from needle-stick injuries not reported.

Sharma, Gilson, Nathan, and Makary (2009), who reported on the incidence of needle-stick injuries in medical school, examined reporting behaviors related to these needle-stick injuries. The study consisted of recent medical school graduates enrolled at surgery residences at 17 medical centers. For 699 respondents, 59 percent reported that they had sustained a needle-stick injury as a medical student, with the median number of needle-stick injuries per respondent being 2.

Of 89 residents who sustained their most recent needle-stick injury during medical school, 47 percent never reported their injury to the employee health office. Why would the residents not report their injury? Underreporting is usually a reflection of the work environment's culture.

Nurses also underreport needle sticks. The American Nurses Association's (ANA) 2008 *Study of Nurses' Views on Workplace Safety and Needle Stick Injuries* reported on an independent survey consisting of more than 700 U.S. nurses. Almost two thirds of nurses reported being accidentally stuck by a needle while at work. Although 86 percent of the nurses reported that their department strongly encouraged reporting of needle-stick injuries, nearly 74 percent of nurses reported that needle sticks go unreported. The two top reasons why nurses felt needle sticks were underreported related to a perception of low risk for infection and the lengthy time to complete the report.

FATIGUE IN THE WORKPLACE

Another area of concern relates to residency training of physicians and their required working hours. How vigilant can health care professionals be to their surroundings when the environment in which they work creates fatigue or stress or both?

The Accreditation Council for Graduate Medical Education (ACGME) approved 2011 standards regarding resident training.

Effective July, 2011, resident dugy hours are limited to 80 hours per week, averaged over a four week time period and includes all in-house call activities and all moonlighting. Residents have to be scheduled for a minimum of one day free every week. With such standards, the duty periods for first-year residents will be limited to not more than 16 hours per 24 hours (ACGME, 2011).

In counterpoint comes the cost of implementation that Nuckols, Bhattacharya, Miller, Ulmer, and Escarce (2009) estimated at $1.6 billion (in 2006 U.S. dollars) across all of the ACGME-accredited programs (with a range of $1.1 to $2.5 billion in sensitivity analysis).

They also concluded that, if the recommendations are highly effective, they could prevent patient harm at reduced or no cost from the societal perspective, despite the fact that the effectiveness of implementation in relation to decreasing medical errors is not known. Not surprisingly, net costs would still remain high for teaching hospitals.

There has been extensive research in the area of resident fatigue and medical errors. A study by West, Tan, Habermann, Sloan, and Shanafelt (2009) examined data from 380 of 430 eligible residents (88.3 percent) at Mayo Clinic, Rochester, Minnesota. This was a prospective longitudinal cohort study where the respondents reported making at least one major medical error during the study period. This study emphasized that fatigue and distress are independently associated with self-perceived medical errors.

Nurses are not immune from fatigue either. Twelve-hour shifts and overtime have become routine to accommodate the current nursing shortage and to fill the holes in shift coverage—the latter having become a tradition though without much thought given to the consequences for patient safety. Mandatory overtime had to become a workplace advocacy issue for the ANA and a legislative issue before hospitals would change the practice.

Brown et al. (2010) reported that sleep deprivation is a common occurrence for nurses working 12-hour shifts, which potentially reduces effectiveness by decreasing their vigilance. They studied 80 registered nurses who were working 3 successive 12-hour shifts (either day or night).

They reported that total sleep time between 12-hour shifts was short (mean 5.5 hours). They concluded that the achieved sleep by nurses working 12-hour shifts is too short and related to increased lapses of attention.

This is consistent with Rogers, Hwang, Scott, Aiken, and Dinges (2004), who randomly sampled 393 registered nurses from a nationwide set of 4,320 members of the ANA. Spiral-bound logbooks were used to collect information about hours worked, time of day worked, overtime, days off, and sleep/wake patterns. Data from the logbooks with demographic questionnaires were summarized using descriptive statistics and frequency tables.

The authors concluded that the risks of making an error were significantly increased when work shifts exceeded 12 hours, when nurses worked overtime, or when they worked more than 40 hours per week.

WORKPLACE SAFETY

Safety in the workplace in health care is a growing concern as well. The Occupational Safety and Health Administration (OSHA) cited the Bureau of Labor Statistics (BLS) report where there were 69 homicides in health services from 1996 to 2000. In 2000, 48 percent of all nonfatal injuries from occupational assaults and violent acts occurred in health care and social services (OSHA, 2004).

Most of these events occurred in hospitals, nursing and personal care facilities, and residential care services. The groups suffering the most from nonfatal assaults resulting in injury were nurses, aides, orderlies, and attendants.

The injury rate patterns indicated that health care and social service groups were at high risk of violent assault at work. The BLS rates measured the number of events per 10,000 full-time workers. The overall health service workers had an incidence rate of 9.3 for injuries resulting from assaults and violent acts in 2000.

The incidence rate for injuries resulting from assaults and violent acts in 2000 for social service workers was much higher at 15, and even higher for nurses and personal care facility workers at 25. This compares to a private sector injury rate of only 2.

More disturbing was the likely fact that incidents of violence in the workplace are underreported, making a true assessment difficult. Nonetheless, in terms of work-related assaults, OSHA reported the following risk factors:

- The accessibility of handguns and other weapons among the patients, families, and/or friends
- The increasing use of hospitals by police and the criminal justice system for criminal holds and the care of acutely disturbed and violent individuals

- The increasing number of acute and chronically mentally ill patients who are being released from hospitals without any follow-up care
- The availability of drugs or money at hospitals or clinics, making them robbery targets
- Unrestricted movement of the public in hospitals and clinics, long waiting times in emergency rooms that lead to client frustration over the inability to provide prompt services
- The increasing presence of gang members, drug or alcohol abusers, trauma patients, or distraught family members
- Low staffing levels during times of increased activities such as mealtimes, visiting times, or during times when patients are transported
- Patient examinations or treatments in isolated work areas.
- Solo work areas with no backup or method to get emergency assistance when needed
- Lack of trained staff who recognize and can effectively manage escalating hostile or assaultive behavior

SPECIALIZATION AND SILOS OF CARE

The American Board of Medical Specialties (ABMS) currently certifies more than 145 specialties and subspecialties (ABMS, 2010). The heterogeneity of physician specialties makes standardization of protocols difficult to implement. Patients are frequently cared for by body part instead of holistically. Because there are so many specialists providing care, communication and coordination becomes increasingly complex.

Therefore, when a patient arrives in the hospital with three or more comorbidities (e.g., diabetes, congestive heart failure, and hypertension) and requires orthopedic surgery such as a hip replacement, the stage is set for potential medical errors to occur, most often due to communication flaws during transition points of care.

WORKPLACE COMMUNICATION

Example 1: A nurse is working in the intensive care unit at a small community hospital in the South. She states that some of the nurses are very reluctant to phone a certain physician, even if the patient's condition warrants it because they are fearful of the certainty of verbal abuse. She goes on to tell that she once called this physician late at night to inform him of his patient's changing condition, only to be told not to bother him again, and then hearing the sharp click of the phone hanging up.

> I called my nursing supervisor because we have a cascade when these events occur. The nursing supervisor called the attending and I received needed orders for this patient but nothing happened to the physician who refused to listen to me.

Example 2: A new graduate nurse says that when she was in nursing school, she cared for only two patients at a time; now she cares for five patients who require total care. "We were taught holistic care in school and spent time getting to know our patients' needs and having meaningful, therapeutic conversations with them. I graduate and find that they just want a waitress; someone to push pills, do baths, do rounds, and document everything, everywhere. The physicians come on the floor and expect us to drop whatever tasks we are doing and assist them immediately. Some of the physicians are just plain rude. The other day one yelled at me because I did not know how to assist with a lumbar puncture; I did not get experience with that procedure in nursing school. I feel pressured all of the time to just get through the shift. This is not why I went into nursing."

The medical group is based on hierarchy, as is nursing. There are physician residents, then chief residents, then attending physicians, and so on up the chain to the chief of staff. There are new nursing graduates, assistant charge nurses, charge nurses, head nurses, nursing supervisors, assistant nursing directors, and the nursing director. Some hospitals encourage extreme stratification of physicians' status by providing special parking spaces, special dining rooms, special treatment, and a reluctance to handle disruptive behaviors.

Other professions also experience disruptive behaviors: pharmacists, ancillary staff, and administrative staff.

In a survey of over 2,000 health care providers by the Institute for Safe Medicine Practices (ISMP) in 2004, 88 percent of respondents encountered condescending language or voice intonation, and 79 percent experienced reluctance or a refusal to answer questions or phone calls. Also, almost half (49 percent) of all respondents told ISMP that their past experiences had altered the way they handle order clarifications or questions about medication orders.

HOW THE WORK ENVIRONMENT AFFECTS NURSING STAFF?

A nationwide study conducted by AMN Healthcare for 5,000 respondents (2010) reported that almost half of the nurses (46 percent) surveyed agreed with the statement, "I worry this job is affecting my health." Also, nearly half of the nurses (44 percent) stated they plan to make a career change in the next 1 to 3 years.

The Joint Commission (2008) acknowledged that intimidating and disruptive behaviors could contribute to medical errors, poor patient satisfaction, and preventable adverse outcomes that increase the cost of care. It initiated two leadership requirements that were implemented in 2009. There must be a code of conduct that actually defines acceptable, disruptive, and inappropriate behaviors. The leaders must develop and implement a process for how they respond and *manage* disruptive and inappropriate behaviors. These standards are integrated into the medical staff requirements and the core competencies in the area of interpersonal skills. The American Organization of Nurse Executives (AONE) and the American College of Physician Executives (ACPE) (2006) published *Guiding Principles for Excellence in Nurse/Physician Relationships*, which stated that at the leadership level, rewards, recognition, and celebration are necessary to promote the behaviors that enhance the nurse/physician relationships within the work environment. This work is embedded within a "just culture" environment and there is a zero tolerance for staff who do not adhere to a code of conduct. The *Guiding Principles* provide a framework to promote interdisciplinary collaboration, respect, and excellent nurse–physician relationships, and a copy is available at http://net.acpe.org/services/AONE/Index.html.

NURSING STAFFING ISSUES

Nursing has also branched out its specialties to align with physician specialties. Nurses specialize in various settings and patient populations. The main difference between the two professions is that, unlike physicians, nurses may be required to work temporarily in areas in which they do not feel competent to provide care.

Therefore, a nurse who works on a general ward may be floated to the intensive care unit for a shift and told that he or she will be assigned the most stable patients. A nurse who works on an adult medical floor may be floated and assigned to care for a pediatric patient. There is also wide variation in how floating practices are monitored in hospitals.

Floating is only one area of concern for safe nurse staffing. The AHRQ (2004) reported on one of the largest studies that examined the records of 5 million medical patients treated at 799 hospitals in 1993. This study reported that medical patients had lower rates of five adverse patient outcomes (urinary tract infections, pneumonia, shock, upper-gastrointestinal bleeding, and prolonged hospital stays) when there was high registered nurse staffing.

When there was high registered nurse staffing, surgery patients had lower rates of urinary tract infections and failure to rescue. Higher rates of nurse staffing were associated with a 3 to 12 percent decrease in adverse outcomes, and higher staffing levels for all levels of nursing staff were associated with a 2 to 25 percent decrease in adverse outcomes, depending on which outcome was studied (AHRQ, 2004).

Aiken et al. (2010) reported that since September of 2009, 14 states and the District of Columbia had passed legislation and/or adopted regulations that addressed nurse staffing, along with another 17 states that were introducing legislation related to nurse staffing.

California was the first state to implement legislation for minimum nurse–patient ratios in 2004. Aiken looked at primary survey data from 22,336 staff nurses within California, Pennsylvania, and New Jersey in 2006 along with the state's hospital discharge databases. The report concluded that hospital nurse staffing ratios that were mandated in California were associated with a lower mortality rate and nurse outcomes predictive of better nurse retention in California and states where the same ratios occur.

The ANA (2010) recently introduced the Registered Nurse Safe Staffing Act of 2010 (S.349/H.R.5227) in response to continued short staffing issues across the United States. This bill would require hospitals to establish committee structures with at least 55 percent direct care nurses or their representatives to serve on the committee.

The committee would be tasked with developing unit-specific nurse staffing plans based on the census, acuity, experience, and skill level of the registered nurses, the availability of support staff to perform non-nursing tasks, and the use of technology. The staffing plan must have adjustable minimum numbers of registered nurses per unit (ANA, 2010).

Various nursing models utilize nursing assistants and licensed practical nurses who work with the registered nurse to provide care for a group of patients. There is wide variation on how these nursing teams communicate with each other when tasks are delegated and monitored by the registered nurse.

I can remember working on a shift long ago where the team leader forgot to assign one of the patients to anyone. It was not until the patient complained half-way through the shift that the error was brought to light and corrected.

Nursing also has opportunities to improve other systems so that more time can be spent at the patient's bedside.

Nurses spend the majority of their time at the nurses station performing activities related to care coordination and documentation. The lack of nurses' time at the bedside combined with other stressors in the work environment creates dissatisfaction among nurses, particularly new nurses. New graduates were identified as a high-risk group for leaving their jobs to seek employment elsewhere.

In a study that was funded by the Robert Wood Johnson Foundation (RWJF) in 2009, lead researcher Linda Honan Pellico analyzed survey comments from 612 new graduate nurses from 34 states and the District of Columbia. The study reported that many new nurses were dissatisfied with their first job. The dissatisfaction was due to numerous unexpected situations in which the new nurses found themselves when employed primarily by hospitals. Approximately 18 percent of new registered nurses were leaving their first nursing employer within only 1 year of starting their job and about 26.2 percent left within 2 years. These nurses reported that pressure to do paperwork meant having to hurry through work and tasks and was not congruent with what they were taught in nursing school (RWJF, 2009).

CONCLUSIONS

Health care is complex, fragmented, and not reliable. Health care organizations need to evaluate their culture, organizational architecture, and communication patterns to search for revision of the current system design to develop and maintain effective patient safety cultures. At times physicians and nurses know the right thing to do, yet they do not do it.

HROs have a reluctance to simplify, are preoccupied with failure, defer to expertise, and are resilient in nature. At the present time, health care organizations in general have a reliability of 10^{-1}, which means that 1 patient out of 10 does not receive the treatment as intended.

In summary, health care is not even reliable in safety for its own workers. How can health care be an HRO without addressing workplace issues for staff?

When staff are fatigued and/or stressed, or fearful of safety in their job, what kind of care can we expect them to provide to patients? Also, when there are poor physician–nurse relationships, the risk of medical error increases due to dysfunctional communication patterns.

How much confidence can the public have that health care's high-risk processes perform consistently every time? When the public flies, they feel pretty safe because aviation has greatly progressed in safety records, whereas health care has not progressed to the same degree and patients are still at risk when care is provided.

It is essential that workflow processes be designed in a manner that makes the work environment safer for physicians and nurses to provide care.

REFERENCES

Accreditation Council for Graduate Medical Education. (2011). Approved standards developed by the ACGME. Retrieved 18 October, 2011, from http://acgme-2010standards.org

Agency for Healthcare Research and Quality. (2004, March). *Research in action: Hospital nurse staffing and quality of care.* AHRQ Publication No. 04-0029. Retrieved June 29, 2010, from http://www.ahrq.gov/research/

Agency for Healthcare Research and Quality. (2008). Transforming hospitals into high reliability organizations. In *Becoming a high reliability organization: Operational advice for hospital leaders.* AHRQ Publication No. 08-0222. Retrieved 19 October, 2011, from http://www.ahrq.gov/qual/hroadvice/

Agency for Healthcare Research and Quality. (n.d.). *Patient safety primer: Teamwork training.* Retrieved January 11, 2011, from http://www.psnet.ahrq.gov/primer.aspx?primerID=8

Aiken, L. H., Sloane, D. M., Cimiotti, J. P., Clarke, S. P., Flynn, L., Seago, J. A., et al. (2010). Implications of the California nurse staffing mandate for other states. *Health services research.* Retrieved January, 12, 2011, from http://www.nursing.upenn.edu/chopr/Documents/Aiken.2010.CaliforniaStaffingRatios.pdf

American Board of Medical Specialties. (2010, June 30). *Physicians participating in ABMS MOC share their stories.* Retrieved 28 June 2010, from http://www.abms.org/News_and_Events/Media_Newsroom/Releases/release_PhysiciansShareMOCStories_063010.aspx

American College of Physician Executives and American Organization of Nurse Executives. (2006). *ACPE and AONE team up to tackle disruptive behavior.* Retrieved June 14, 2010, from http://net.acpe.org/services/AONE/Index.html

AMN Healthcare. (2010). *Survey of registered nurses: Job satisfaction and career plans.* Retrieved June 14, 2010, from http://www.amnhealthcare.com/News/staffing-matters-details.aspx?Id=33432

American Nurses Association. (2008). *2008 study of nurses' views on workplace safety and needle stick injuries.* Retrieved January 11, 2011, from http://www.nursingworld.org/MainMenuCategories/Occupationaland Environmental/occupationalhealth/OccupationalResources/2008Safety andNeedlestickStudy.aspx

American Nurses Association. (2010, July 7). *Registered nurse safe staffing bill introduced in congress: Direct care nurses would drive staffing plans to ensure patient safety.* Retrieved June 29, 2010, from http://www.nursingworld .org/safestaffingbill

Brown, G., Rogers, J., Bausell, R., Trinkoff, A., Kane, R., & Scharf, S. M. (2010). Lapses of attention and reaction time in sleep deprived nurses working successive 12-hour shifts. *Journal of Sleep and Sleep Disorders Research, 33,* Abstract 0295.

Hickner, J., Graham, D. G., Elder, N. C., Brandt, E., Emsermann, C. B., Dovey, S., et al. (2007). Testing process errors and their harms and consequences reported from family medicine practices: A study of the American Academy of Family Physicians National Research Network. *Quality and Safety in Health Care, 17*(3), 194–200.

Institute for Safe Medicine Practices. (2004). *Medication safety alert: Intimidation: Practitioners speak up about this unresolved problem. Part I.* Retrieved June 10, 2010, from http://www.ismp.org/newsletters/acutecare/articles/20040311_2.asp

Johns Hopkins Medicine. (2009, March 11). *Diagnostic errors: The new focus of patient safety experts.* Retrieved July 30, 2010, from http://www.hopkins medicine.org/news/media/releases/diagnostic_errors_the_new_ focus_of_patient_safety_experts

Joint Commission. (2008, July). *Sentinel event alert: Behaviors that undermine a culture of safety.* Retrieved January 12, 2011, from http://docs.google .com/viewer?a=v&q=cache:21pzbtgNxT0J:www.jointcommission .org/assets/1/18/SEA_40.PDF+joint+commission+requirements+ disruptive+behavior&hl=en&gl=us&pid=bl&srcid=ADGEESjfndlf633 hzkdWICAM2DnWBAnjGkhfAt5RM8s8xUGy7KNHBcziiYo2F4f 7giPiFgGqAakuXvwLKAGkB5R06uSXX4U81EBwKjWUVjXB__LPgKP QFlqE1AwlNnONNtSpFB41S0Ov&sig=AHIEtbRqbyubvCXqMOetacDI KCxiJvIhLQ

Newman-Toker, D.E., Provonost, P.J., (March, 2009) Commenatries: Diagnostic errors-The next frontier for patient safety. *Journal American Medical Association, 30*(10), 1060.

Nolan, T., Resar, R. Haraden, C., & Griffin, F. A. (2004). *Improving the reliability of health care.* IHI Innovation Series white paper. Retrieved July 30, 2010, from http://www.ihi.org/IHI/Results/WhitePapers/ ImprovingtheReliabilityofHealthCare.htm

Nuckols, T. K., Bhattacharya, J., Miller, D., Ulmer, C., & Escarce, J. J. (2009). Cost implications of reduced work hours and workloads for resident physicians. *The New England Journal of Medicine, 360*, 2202–2215.

Occupational Safety and Health Administration. (2004). *Guidelines for preventing workplace violence for health care & social service workers.* OSHA 3148-01R 2004. Retrieved 30 July, 2010, from http://www.osha.gov/Publications/OSHA3148/osha3148.html

Perrow, C. (1984). *Normal accidents: Living with high-risk technologies. New York:* Basic Books.

Roberts, K. H. (n.d.). *HRO has prominent history.* Retrieved July 30, 2010, from http://www.apsf.org/newsletters/html/2003/spring/hrohistory.htm

Rogers, A. E., Hwang, W. T., Scott, L. D., Aiken, L. H., & Dinges, D. F. (2004). The working hours of hospital staff nurses and patient safety. *Health Affairs, 23*(4), 202–212.

Robert Wood Johnson Foundation. (2009). *Understanding and preventing departures: Surprises in work environment contribute to high turnover rates of new nurses.* Retrieved August 20, 2010, http://www.rwjf.org/pr/product.jsp?id=46437

Sharma, G. K., Gilson, M. M., Nathan, H., & Makary, M. (2009). Needlestick injuries among medical students: Incidence and implications. *Academic Medicine, 84*(12), 1815–1821.

West, C. P., Tan, A. D., Habermann, T. M., Sloan, J. A., & Shanafelt, T. D. (2009). Association of resident fatigue and distress with perceived medical errors. *JAMA, 302*(12), 1294–1300.

Wilson, B., Miler, K., Wong, B., Emmons R., MacDonald, K., Martin, P., et al. (2005b). *Improvement report: Improving hand hygiene practice with six sigma.* Storyboard presentation at IHI's Natonal Forum. Retrieved January 30, 2011, from http://www.ihi.org/IHI/Topics/PatientSafety/SafetyGeneral/ImprovementStories/ImprovingHandHygienePracticewithSixSigma.htm

7

Organizational Architecture in Relation to Accreditation and Patient Safety Efforts: Ready, Fire, Aim

ACCREDITATION AND ORGANIZATIONAL ARCHITECTURE

IOM described the attributes for the ideal health care system, but did not provide the requirements for the organizational architecture that might best lead to health care there.

The Joint Commission does not offer much in the way of organizational architecture either. There is, most likely, not one path to follow but many, depending on the characteristics of the organization's values and goals.

Here is an experience worth noting in this regard. I once sat with a well-educated patient who wanted to share his dissatisfaction regarding his hospital stay with someone. This is what I remember him saying

> I hate hospitals. What is it about you people? From the minute I arrived, I was dehumanized by being provided a gown that stripped me of any perceived dignity I might have left—with the gaps open and flapping behind me for the world to see my backside.

I am a capable person in my home where I take my own medications and eat and sleep when I want. Seems I am now an incompetent old man who has to have his medications controlled and delivered by a nurse. I have lost my right to eat when I am hungry, take a nap at my leisure or have a stroll around the grounds just to breathe in some fresh air.

The only thing I could do at that time was listen to his concerns and have his wife bring him his pajamas.

Clearly, health care is not patient centered and frequently not effective or safe.

Senge's work on systems, however, emphasizes that "structure shapes behavior." Organizational architecture either enhances the work or hinders the work. It involves the framework that guides the daily behaviors related to how the work gets done.

According to Nadler, Tushman, and Nadler (1997), information technology is transforming the work environment. The traditional constraints related to geographic locations no longer exist. Information can reach all workers simultaneously; this also eliminates the need for unnecessary levels of bureaucracy that were created to handle flow of information.

Alignment of the formal and informal structures with tasks and people are essential for effective organizational architecture. In fact, alignment is key to strategy and relationships. Relationships form and inform us, and those relationships start at the top.

Another advantage made possible by technology concerns the use of teams; this involves using staff as human capital to best engage their collective knowledge, expertise, creativity, and judgment when multitasking, and creating thereby a more flexible workforce.

In turn, a new set of leadership skills is required, with increased autonomy provided to every level of the organization. Clearly, when informal work groups are not in agreement with strategic plans, staff resistance can make it very difficult for the organization to sustain or attain successful levels of patient care.

As such, strategic plans need to be congruent with external forces and internal forces; otherwise, they will not succeed in the long haul. The higher the degree of resources that an organization has, the more the options for strategic choices.

The Joint Commission's standards for the medical staff require that the medical staff work with the governing body and administration in a collaborative fashion and agree together on how to accomplish their work (Joint Commission, 2011).

In addition, the Joint Commission leadership standards provide leaders with increasing accountability to evaluate their culture of safety and quality on a regular basis and prioritize and implement changes identified by that evaluation (Joint Commission, 2009). It also outlined expectations for a code of conduct that spells out what acceptable behavior is and how leadership will handle disruptive or inappropriate behaviors.

The organizational architecture is frequently a source of underlying causes for workplace issues. As stated earlier, all organizational structures have the capacity either to enhance or to hinder the work.

The Location of the Work Enhances or Hinders the Work

The location and organization of offices, design of patient rooms, laboratories, and ancillary staff services either enhance or hinder the work. The traditional, centralized nursing station hub, for example, creates several problems that increase possibility of errors, including high traffic flow with noise and distractions.

One example of this is a hospital that had a large medical floor. Here, the acuity of patients had crept up until it was clear that a step-down unit with telemetry capability was needed for higher acuity patients. The workflow, formerly and exclusively centralized around the nurse station, was changed. Decentralized hubs were developed to decrease traffic flow at the central nurse station, enabling the placement of patients' medical records near those patients. The result is that these simple changes largely enhanced the workflow process.

Hospital Committees Enhance or Hinder the Work

Hospital committees carry out the board's directives and drive patient safety and quality efforts; however, many such committees are outdated and dysfunctional. When the flow of information is slow or nonexistent, it hinders patient safety and accreditation efforts.

Hospital committees also endure the hazard of being "siloed" with little to no cross-communication between committees. For example, if there is an environmental issue that requires follow-up by the Infection Control Committee, how does that information flow from the group handling the environmental issue to the Infection Control Committee and how long does it take to get on the Infection Control Committee's agenda?

Many years ago, I sat on a few committees where, as they say, "the minutes were taken and the hours were wasted." As some of these committees required no preparation on my part, I asked a committee chairman what my expected role for committee participation was. The response is that I should attend ad hoc when needed.

Committees require a charter that becomes their mission statement. The charter tells why the committees exist and what they are "charged" to do. All committee members have a defined role. There can be subcommittees that are working groups or the committee (if not too large) can itself be the working group.

Representation on committees by patients seems logical because the patient is the key stakeholder and the reason why the organization exists in the first place. Yet, many health care organizations do not have patients serve on committees.

At the board level, sometimes patients' needs get lost in the sea of statistics that are presented at high-level board meetings. It is important for board members to always be aware that their work is linked to patients and their families and that patients' lives are influenced by each number on the quality and patient safety dashboard. In this light, the Institute for Healthcare Improvement's (IHI, n.d.) recommendation that storytelling be used as a method to keep board members engaged in quality and patient safety efforts is a good one.

Nursing Models Enhance or Hinder the Work

Functional Nursing Model

Functional nursing is a care model that calls to mind work patterns in manufacturing. Nursing assignments are given by functions: one nurse passes all medications, one nurse does all treatments, and one nursing assistant or licensed practical nurse does vital signs and/or patient baths. This nursing care delivery system is task oriented.

According to Robinson (n.d.), functional nursing was the norm for U.S. hospitals in the late 1800s and through the end of World War II. Hospitals were searching for more efficient methods to reduce labor costs. The focus was on completing the tasks of the day, not on holistic patient care. This was an efficient model but not necessarily an effective one for nurse and patient satisfaction. With the functional model, it is easy for patients' needs to get lost in the emphasis on the performance of tasks.

As a nursing student, I worked in a large metropolitan teaching hospital as a nursing technician—a terminology used then. In that role, I was assigned all the treatments and vital signs on the floor—a 35-bed mixed medical/surgical floor. Between doing vital signs and treatments, I also replenished the ice water containers for the patients in each room. I had documented the vital signs on a clipboard, which I then transcribed into the medical record along with my observations from the treatments. Anything out of the norm was reported to the registered nurse.

Team Nursing Model

Team nursing uses just the team that includes the registered nurse as the leader of the team, licensed practical nurses, and nurse aides. The team leader is assigned a group of patients for whom they will provide care during the shift. Team nursing makes use of each team member's competencies in caring for a group of patients.

The licensed practical nurse (LPN) may give medications and perform treatments; the nurse aide assists with baths, transport, and vital signs; and the registered nurse may perform the assessments, patient education, and coordination of the care.

Huber (2000), in his overview of history for the various types of nursing care delivery models, described team nursing as follows:

Team nursing was established in the early 1950s because of the dissatisfaction with functional nursing. The risk point for team nursing lies in the skill set of the team leader.

Team nursing can be very effective. Again, many hospitals assumed that nurses had the proper skill set to handle being team leaders. In fact, there was, and still is, wide variation in team performance.

If there are clear roles and communication patterns, and consistent behaviors of respect and collegiality by team members who continually learn how to work together better as a team, then team nursing can work very well. If the roles are not defined well and the team does not even know how to be a team, then team nursing does not work very well. This can lead to increased conflict due to role ambiguity and poor communication. Also, due to costs, many hospitals dilute the team leader's role. Ideally, the team leader does not have a patient assignment. He or she is responsible for the whole group of patients. He or she does rounds, assessments, and coordinates with other disciplines to navigate the complexity of the system for that shift and serves as mentor for the team members.

Modular Nursing Model

Modular nursing started in the 1980s, when hospital design was spatially oriented to caring for clusters of patients in geographic zones. These zones provided for decentralization of care, with some zones called pods. The zones were typically stocked with linen, supplies, and medications. Nurses were assigned to a zone to care for a group of patients.

Primary Nursing Model

Primary nursing began in the 1970s, again due to dissatisfaction with functional and team models that still did not live up to holistic care. With primary care, there can be increased accountability at the bedside. Usually, the registered nurse is partnered with an "extender" with varying capabilities.

Patient-Focused Care Model

Parsley and Corrigan (1999) stated that the term "patient-focused care" is attributed to the work accomplished at the Lakeland Medical Center in Florida that started in 1988. The key difference in this model is that cross-training and multiskilling is done, so that there is increased flexibility in the performance of role functions. Nurses may do electrocardiograms (EKGs), perform respiratory therapy treatments, draw blood, and so forth. The inpatient, outpatient, diagnostic, and therapeutic services are grouped together in one location and patients who have similar diagnoses and needs are grouped in another.

The registered nurse may still be the team leader. The goal is for caregivers to provide up to 80 percent of the care that patients need without the patient leaving the nursing unit. This is a radical change in delivery of care that substantially reconfigures roles in providing care to patients. There are also changes in altered reporting relationships as well as physical remodeling for unit-based pharmacies, laboratories, supplies, and unit-based admissions and discharges.

According to Parsley and Corrigan, multiskilling and cross-training were the most controversial elements of patient-focused care.

Jennings (2008) reviewed care models for AHRQ and concluded that, despite the variety of care models noted, there has been no rigorous evaluation across models regarding their effectiveness toward enhanced patient safety.

This means that to date we know very little about the relationship between nursing care delivery models and patient safety. Also, the ability to collect longitudinal data for evaluation is difficult within the rapidly changing health care environment.

Kane, Shamliyan, Mueller, Duval, and Wilt (2007) provided a report on nurse staffing and quality of patient care to AHRQ. They reviewed observational studies that examined the relationship between nurse staffing and outcomes. Classes of patients and hospital characteristics were separately analyzed.

Results indicated that increased registered nurse staffing was associated with decreased hospital mortality, failure to rescue, cardiac arrest, hospital-acquired pneumonia, and other adverse events. The impact of increased registered nurse staffing on patient outcomes was consistent for intensive care units and for surgical patients. Greater overtime hours worked were associated with an increase in hospital-related mortality, nosocomial infections, shock, and bloodstream infections.

The researchers could find no studies that directly examined the factors that influence nurse-staffing policy, and few studies evaluated the role of agency staff on patient outcomes.

In the end, they concluded that greater nurse staffing was associated with better outcomes in intensive care units and in surgical patients. Also, increased nurse staffing in hospitals was associated with lower hospital-related mortality, failure to rescue, and other patient outcomes; however, the association is not necessarily causal. Estimates of the nursing effect size has to be adjusted by characteristics of providers. This includes hospital commitment to high quality care which is not even considered in most studies.

Documentation Systems Enhance or Hinder the Work

According to a time and motion study conducted by Hendrich, Chow, Skierczynski, and Lu (2008), nurses spend 35.3 percent of their time documenting care of patients. Clearly, documentation is an area to explore for devising ways to obtain greater efficiency for nurses, so that they can spend more time caring for patients.

I have worked in hospitals where the nurse had to document the identical piece of information in at least three different places. Redundancy in documentation wastes nursing time. I have also seen basic tasks documented in the nurses' notes when use of flow sheets would suffice. Care paths may be used and supplemented with flow sheets for documentation of routine care.

If the team meets and discusses the plan of care for the day, then everyone, including the patient, knows what is expected for the day. Documentation would include the patient's response to the care provided, be integrated with all disciplines, and include the patient's comments as well. Because I think this is important, I used to provide a note pad to all of my patients and sit with them to write out questions for the physician.

Typically, if this is not done, the patient forgets to ask because he or she is either stressed, in pain, and/or fatigued. Also, physicians spend only a few minutes with each patient as they make their rounds. Patients should be allowed to write their questions directly in the medical record as part of their participation in their health care.

Staff Evaluations Enhance or Hinder the Work

Every year, most health care organizations evaluate their employees' performance; however, there is minimal or zero linkage between performance and participation on teams.

If the hospital values teamwork, then participation on teams should be integrated into the evaluation system; the same goes for quality and patient safety.

Team evaluation would provide an opportunity for the staff member to see himself or herself through the various lenses of the other team members as well as through the measurement of outcomes achieved by the team. This type of feedback also could be very useful in building high-performing teams at the unit level.

Physician and Patient Safety: Cultural Competencies Enhance or Hinder the Work

An operating room nurse tells about the surgeon's initial reactions to the time-out procedure that has to be done as part of the requirements for accreditation: "We had the chief of surgery saying he was not going to do it. He thought it was a big waste of time and silly. Wrong site surgery would never happen to him or his colleagues. The chief of staff had to get involved and send a clear message that implementation was not optional."

A quality specialist who trains physicians how to perform root cause analysis shares her story:

> Sometimes, it is difficult. I have worked with physicians who tried to conduct root cause analysis in the same way that they perform peer review. They tended to want to look at the "who" rather than the "why" and "how."

Physicians are key stakeholders in patient safety. Recently, the NPSF published the Lucian Leape Institute Roundtable on Reforming Medical Education report (2010), which concluded that although there is substantial improvement in patient safety, much more needs to be done. The report's recommendations centered along three common themes:

Medical schools and teaching hospitals need to emphasize patient safety, along with model professionalism. They need to encourage transparency and collaborative behaviors and have zero tolerance for egregiously disrespectful or abusive behavior.

Medical schools should teach patient safety as a basic science and also teach interpersonal and communication skills through experiences in teams with other health care professionals.

Medical schools and teaching hospitals need to launch intensive faculty development programs so that faculty have the requisite knowledge and skills to permit them to effectively function as teachers and as role models for students.

Nursing and Patient Safety: Cultural Competencies Enhance or Hinder the Work

Benner, Sutphen, Leonard, and Day (2009) reported that today's nurses do not have enough education to meet the demands of practice. They concluded that the present nursing education structure is inadequate for the current complexity required to care for patients and their families. This study did not include patient safety as a recommended science but did say that nursing programs need to do better in teaching nursing science, natural sciences, social sciences, technology, and the humanities.

The American Association of Colleges of Nursing (AACN, 2006) convened a task force and organized core competencies to selected categories of the conceptual framework that is used in the Essentials of Baccalaureate Education of Professional Nursing Practice.

Patient safety is integrated into the core competencies of critical thinking, health care systems and policy, communication, illness and disease management, ethics, and information and health care technologies. One example of this integration is related to essential communication recommendations.

The nurse is to establish and maintain effective working relationships and open communication and cooperation from the interdisciplinary team. Also, the nurse is to always use a standardized approach to "hand off" communications, including an opportunity to ask and respond to questions.

Another example relates to ethics in nurses' daily practice: The nurse will take action to prevent or to limit unsafe or unethical health and nursing care practices by others.

Health care professionals generally agree with Lucian Leape that patient safety concepts need to be taught as a science in nursing, medical, and other health care professionals' schools, but the question remains, "Then what?"

If the new graduate does not find congruence with what he or she has been taught in school and then enters the workplace where hierarchy and status are seemingly more important than the patient's safety, then the health care professional will most likely leave the organization—or worse, will accommodate new, unhealthy behaviors to maintain his or her job.

Ready, Fire, Aim

I once toured a hospital that had several different buildings ranging from very old construction to new construction. Some of the buildings had been linked by stairways; other buildings required a walk outside to get to your final destination. Each building looked entirely different than the one adjacent to it. Some of the floors were old and chipped; some of the floors were new and shiny. The layout reminded me of a giant jigsaw puzzle for which there had been no final plan or picture of what the end product should look like. It was evident that short planning cycles had been performed in a crisis mode and without a vision of what the future might hold for those, and perhaps other, areas.

Patient safety and accreditation are not programs to be built on cycles of activity without a vision of what the future might hold. The best architectural design needs to be congruent with a vision of the future.

Clearly, patient safety concepts and behaviors should be integrated into the daily work of frontline staff. Many of the accreditation standards are patient safety related and, as such, also need to be integrated into the daily work of frontline staff. Not utilizing a systems approach in organizational planning when developing patient safety and accreditation initiatives is analogous to firing a gun without considering the target (the aims of the programs and what the desired goals/outcomes will be).

Some health care organizations implement a patient safety program by initiating a patient safety committee, providing some resources, providing some training on patient safety concepts, and then later wondering if their efforts have been fruitful or if the patient safety program was just one more accreditation requirement. Some health care organizations gear up for their 3-year accreditation cycle in periodic waves of intense activity that slow down considerably, immediately after the year of the accreditation cycle.

Sometimes, the specific aims for patient safety and accreditation do not serve as the basis for guiding the decisional framework for the leadership. For example, organizational priorities often compete and conflict. Quality is not free, neither is patient safety. Both require use of technologies that are expensive to implement and also necessary when designing safer systems of care. Several examples follow:

Example 1: A seasoned nursing supervisor working in a small community hospital says that the hospital's patient safety program is not integrated well and that chronic issues are still not being addressed.

"Nursing staffing is now looked at when root cause analysis is performed as a potential contributing factor; however, we don't see much improvement in that area because we are held to the annual budget requirements."

"We have a policy for disruptive behavior as an accreditation requirement, but these events are not tracked and trended; and staff feels not much is done about them," she said.

When asked about leadership's involvement, the supervisor states that they have an administrator who "caters" to the physicians.

"Physicians are viewed as revenue generating; nurses are viewed as an expense."

"Most staff would not be able to tell you who the administrator is; he seldom makes rounds on the units."

Example 2: Another hospital implemented a patient safety program. The administrator ensured that a patient safety committee was appointed and that there was a patient safety manager who handled the root causes analysis and failure mode and effect analysis projects. The patient safety manager focused on the functions specified in his job. Databases were not integrated so the patient safety manager had to meet on a regular basis with the risk management section to review all incident reports to assess if root cause analysis was needed. He was denied access to the risk management database.

Recently, the patient safety manager was wondering if opportunities are being missed because patterns of events are not integrated centrally into an enterprise database.

Example 3: "Why can't the staff just get along together?" a registered nurse asks who works on a busy medical floor in an urban teaching hospital. "You know nursing has suffered from a high turnover rate for the past 5 years. We just can't keep nurses on this unit. I no sooner train someone then they up and leave. I am tired of doing this extra work in training staff all of the time in addition to my regular duties." The medical floor has 50 beds and has a high acuity level. The nurse to patient ratio is 6:1. The traffic flow on the unit is also high: consultants stream in during peak times in the morning and the afternoon, leaving a trail of orders behind them. "Some of the physicians do not accept being questioned about any orders they write; they become defensive and make you feel stupid for asking them any questions at all," she said.

She tells a story about one of the new nurses in orientation. "Rounds can get confusing here; between the attending and the consultants, plus all of the diagnostic work-ups that are being done . . . and if just one of your patients becomes unstable, the other five suffer and sometimes routine tasks are carried over for the next shift to handle. I know we have a patient safety program, but it seems we don't take enough steps in being proactive with opportunities with near misses. I wish that the administration would make rounds on our unit and listen to us; they might be surprised at how much we really know."

Patient Safety and Quality Concepts

There are similarities and differences in quality and patient safety.

Quality has a special language, as patient safety does. Quality has special tools, as patient safety does. Quality cannot be delegated and neither can patient safety be. Quality is the responsibility of everyone in the organization, so is patient safety. It is not a program; it is a journey toward high reliability, and the leadership has to be engaged and on board to successfully implement a quality or patient safety program. What are the differences?

Organizational architecture involves the design of all of the elements within the system that produces outcomes. This includes the formal and the informal structures within the organization. More importantly, according to Nadler et al. (1992), this includes the design of the work systems and the social systems that are included within the larger and complex organization. When any of the elements within a system are dysfunctional, the entire system will be affected in some manner.

Many times the dysfunctional effects are experienced on the front line of care. I have heard numerous stories in that regard from health care professionals who have experienced either having family members as patients in health care or they themselves required medical treatment. Hospital staff will tell you that physicians and nurses make the worst patients and can be the most troublesome for health care staff when their family members enter the health care system. This is because physicians and nurses know there is risk involved even when only basic care is provided, and they also know the right thing that should be done.

The interactions that patients and families have with health care professionals from the first encounter at admissions to the last encounter in the discharge process determine how they rank the quality received. When the patient and/or their family have a bad experience and suffer harm from an adverse event, the risk of loss of trust, both at the provider level and at the system level, is also present. Once trust is lost, it is extremely difficult to regain.

Because health care is increasingly complex, simple solutions for patient safety will most likely not be effective.

Health care organizations need to use a systems approach to examine the patterns within the organization that dynamically interact with each other on a continuous basis and search for opportunities to make improvements. Health care organizations also need to apply Senge's competencies of systems thinking, mental models, personal mastery, shared vision, and team learning to transform into a learning organization.

We have looked into the mirror and the real enemy of change is ourselves. The medical profession is autonomous and clinically focused. The basic underpinnings of the Hippocratic Oath to "do no harm" resonates in the clinical settings. Staff look for who is to blame when adverse events occur.

When I was a head nurse on an intensive care unit, I recall counseling a nurse for making a medication error that resulted in patient harm. In telling her to "be more careful," I also thought (erroneously) that I had prevented the adverse event from recurring. It is difficult sometimes, for clinicians, who are viewing only their piece of the system, to view events from a holistic perspective.

We know now that the results we see are the product (either intentionally or unintentionally) of system design. The system is perfectly designed to produce its output. As a result, one cannot expect to continue doing the same things and obtain different results. Counseling someone for making a medication error does not change the system that led to him or her making the mistake in the first place. For example, when root cause analysis is done on this event and "why" questions are applied, we find the following dialogue:

Q: Why was the nurse's action considered a medication error?

A: She gave the medication to the wrong patient.

Q: Why did she give the medication to the wrong patient?

A: She had two extra patients that day and one patient was being transferred to the intensive care unit. She admitted she did not perform the usual medication checks.

Q: Why did she have two extra patients?

A: The vacancy rates on this unit are high and coverage with overtime was not possible that day due to staff sick calls.

Q: Why are the vacancy rates high?

A: Recruitment has been difficult.

Q: Why has recruitment been difficult?

A: The salary and benefit package is not congruent with the local market.

Q: Why is the salary and benefit package not congruent with the local market?

A: The budget for this year does not allow matching the salary and benefit package to the local market.

So, with just a few questions, we have traveled from the provider error to faulty system design due to leadership decisions regarding budgetary constraints. It is much easier to punish the staff member and move on quickly; however, that does nothing to correct the faulty system design. In fact, it prevents learning because future mistakes will not be reported when staff are fearful of being punished. So, this logic sets up perpetual system failures.

Basic Concepts of Systems

A system is a collection of subsystems that interact to accomplish an overall goal. This includes inputs, processes, outputs, and outcomes.

The goal of the system is to maximize the output of the system, not the output of each of its components. This requires that each component of the system is optimized, not maximized. According to Reid, Compton, Grossman, and Fanjiang (2005), optimization of the system requires a clear understanding of the whole system as well as the interactions of the subsystems. Optimization also implies that each component is effective and does what it is supposed to do, at the right time, every time. Optimization implies reliability as well as functionality. Health care processes that do not possess high reliability increase the probability for error to occur.

Complex systems and open systems are both at risk of producing unintended consequences. Health care is a complex adaptive system. Rouse (2008) described certain characteristics for them: they are nonlinear and dynamic, resulting in system behaviors that may appear to be random or even chaotic.

At times it is difficult to see the nonlinear patterns due to the passage of time between events. Economists know this. There will be lag time between interest rates cycling up or down and the events that actually caused this to happen. It takes a while before it is clear the country is in a recession; it also takes a while to see improvement in the economy and determine when the country is moving out of the recession.

In health care, time lags between actions and visible consequences can be several years. For example, going back to the example of the nurse who made the medication error, the "why" questions ultimately led to lack of budget money to compete with the local market as a contributing cause. The local market did not change overnight. There was a lag time between the vacancy rates increasing for nurses and the system's response to this.

Each person tends to adapt over time to each other's behaviors. Adaptation and learning result in self-organization. A wide variation of behavior patterns that may spark innovation or unfortunate accidents emerge over time.

Team training teaches staff to have meaningful dialogue where the patient becomes the center of the conversation. There is no place for egos in patient-centered care. Anyone should be able to question any staff member if he or she observes any behavior that might have the potential for patient harm.

There is no single point of control. This means that system behaviors are often unpredictable and uncontrollable. The behaviors are usually more easily influenced than controlled.

The key to designing effective, adaptive, complex systems is to strategize and create the ability to maximize system agility, monitor itself for performance, and take into account stakeholders' input. For example, what kind of outcomes does the system wish to achieve? What are the benefits of these outcomes, to which stakeholders?

How do we know in health care that we are optimizing the domains of quality? For example, effectiveness relies on the best applied knowledge at the time of the intervention, which changes with time. Evidence-based medicine involves making the right day-to-day clinical decisions based on the current best evidence. The right patient receives the right care. There has been an explosion of medical knowledge in the past 10 years.

There is no physician who can rely on his or her memory to integrate all of the information required for day-to-day clinical decision making. Evidence-based medicine is a growing field, with information available for further review at:

National Institutes of Health: www.nih.gov.

The Cochrane Collaboration: www.cochrane.org

Centre for Evidence-Based Medicine: www.cebm.net

According to Schyve (2005), there are certain challenges when systems approaches are applied to health care: each of these challenges requires a different way of thinking by the providers who care for patients.

Deming emphasized giving up looking for the bad apples and ceasing mass inspection. He emphasized building quality into the product in the first place and helping staff to do a better job through continuous learning.

System Aims

The focus of the goal for a system needs to be maximizing the entire system's ability to achieve a particular output, rather than focusing on the output of each component within the system.

Systems comprise multiple, interconnected components: machines, processes, data, and people. The interrelationships are dynamic and continuous and affect each other's performance as well as the system's overall performance. Information informs and forms us.

Patterns of communication enhance or hinder the work. Having the right people communicate using the right data transformed into information enables transfer of learning and increases the probability of making better decisions.

The output of a system has multiple dimensions. In health care, the dimensions of safety, effectiveness, patient-centeredness, timeliness, efficiency, and equity are used for defining the output of the system for optimization; however, the judgment of attaining optimization of each component is value laden depending on the view of the stakeholder.

For example, how do health care professionals know when a system has optimized safety as a dimension? How is the system's success measured?

If safety is defined as "prevention from harm caused inadvertently by health care workers," then it seems reasonable that noting events of preventable patient harm would be reasonable measurements of success. The fewer the number of preventable harmful events that occur, the more effective the safety system is. The IHI has a "Trigger Tool for Measuring Adverse Events," which is offered free for download at www.ihi.org/IHI/Results/WhitePapers/IHIGlobalTriggerToolWhitePaper.htm

Provonost (2010) recently argued that mortality rates should not be the gold standard for quality of care because mortality rates include nonpreventable as well as preventable causes of death. Also, preventable deaths occur only in approximately 1 out of 20 patients in hospitals in the United States.

He further argued that processes such as prevention of central line–associated bloodstream infections should be measured because they are preventable and a zero rate is achievable. Therefore, the system should aim to have zero needless deaths and zero incidents of preventable harm measured on a continuous basis as measurements for safety.

Most systems are dependent upon even larger systems in which they reside and exchange information with on a continuous basis. Most systems are open systems and have continuous and dynamic interactions internally and externally.

All of health care reform and reimbursement structures shape external market forces and drive internal shifts in policy and subsequent behaviors. Accreditation standards shape health care system behaviors that must continually adapt to the new external requirements imposed.

Complex systems and open systems both have risk of producing unintended consequences.

An example of this relates to mandatory performance measures. Bromley and Franklin (2007) reported that Joint Commission and CMS extended the 4-hour window for initial administration of empiric antibiotics for cases of pneumonia to 6 hours of hospital arrival as a result of concerns expressed by the field that potentially unnecessary antibiotic administration might occur.

Cost Considerations

According to Graves (2004), approximately 1 in 10 patients who are admitted to a hospital will acquire an infection that results in substantial economic loss. Estimates of the costs of these infections in 2002 were $6.7 billion in the United States and approximately $1.7 billion in the United Kingdom.

The IOM *First Do No Harm: To Err is Human: Building a Safer Health System* estimated total national costs of preventable adverse events in the United States to be between $17 billion and $29 billion annually, with health care costs representing over one-half of that amount.

A study in 2008 by Mello, Studdert, and Thomas for the Commonwealth Fund tested the extent to which hospitals actually absorb the costs of medical errors. Mello and colleagues did a comparison of the costs, which included malpractice insurance premiums and costs of additional inpatient care that the hospital was not able to recoup by passing on to other payers.

The researchers used data from 14,732 discharge records in Utah and Colorado in 1992. There was an estimated cost of approximately $439 million, and the average cost for negligent injuries was $113,280.

Of the 24 hospitals, 17 passed on 80 percent or more of the costs associated with adverse events, with no significant differences noted between teaching and nonteaching hospitals. Therefore, it was determined by this group that hospitals actually bear just a small proportion of the actual costs for adverse events.

Mello and his group concluded that external incentives, such as the CMS program stopping payment for events that should "never" happen, may provide assistance but are not enough.

Health courts that broaden the scope of claims allowed for patients and also that have reasonable limits set to awards received may provide incentive by directing a larger proportion of the costs of avoidable injuries back to the involved providers along with their insurers.

There is always a business case for doing the right thing for patients, their families, and significant others. Leaders decide on the right thing to do every day and their decisions ripple out and shape the environment in which health care is provided.

It is the right thing to provide a safe working environment for staff; it is the right thing to provide safe care to patients. Processes that have higher reliability translate into safer, more efficient care.

When staff communicate better with each other and with their patients, better outcomes are achieved. When staff can feel that their work has meaning and a greater purpose than just accomplishing the tasks at hand, there is greater worker engagement. Greater worker engagement translates into a lower turnover rate, which saves money spent in recruitment costs, orientation, and replacement of staff during the vacancy period with overtime costs.

Finally, a better practice environment in which egos are checked at the door and everyone has the moral obligation to question any action that may jeopardize patient care without fear of humiliation or reprisal translates into a better and safer workplace culture.

Learning Organization's Core Competencies

Senge's *Fifth Discipline* (1990) outlines five competencies that support a learning organization: systems thinking, mental models, personal mastery, shared vision, and team learning. All of these competencies are necessary to optimize the aims of the system.

Systems thinking: Integrates all of the other disciplines by comprehension of the whole and the interrelationships between the parts.

Mental models: Staff are aware of their view of the world and use inquiry, reflection, and effective communication techniques that enhance meaningful dialogue. These conversations stimulate genuine learning.

Personal mastery: Staff have the ability to continually see their connectedness to the world, with compassion and commitment to the whole. This means that staff know their higher purpose and are committed to it with passion.

Shared vision: Staff can articulate what the system is intended to achieve as the future state for the organization, which translates into a collective consciousness and coherent set of priorities that move the organization forward toward its goals.

Team learning: Staff have the ability to communicate both across and up and down the organizational chart and have meaningful dialogue with team members that improves the team's effectiveness over time.

Patient safety needs to be integrated into the microsystem. A clinical microsystem is defined as "a group of clinician and staff working together with a shared clinical purpose to provide care for a population of patients" (Mohr, Batalden, & Barach, 2004). They cited eight dimensions for high-performing microsystems:

1. Constancy of purpose
2. Investment in improvement

3. Alignment of the roles and training for efficiency and staff satisfaction

4. Reliance on other team members to do the work; recognition of an interdependence of roles to meet patient care needs

5. Integration of information and technology that is embedded into the work flows

6. Continuous measurements of outcomes

7. Supportive environment provided by the larger organization

8. Connection to the community served and extended influence to that sector

Models for Patient Safety

Microsystems

Microsystems consist of a core team of health professions, a defined population of patients or customers for which they provide care, an information environment supportive of the care they provide, and support staff and equipment with an office environment. The goal of a microsystem is "to foster an emphasis on small, replicable, functional service systems that enable front-line staff to provide efficient, excellent and patient-centered care" (Agency for Healthcare Research and Quality [AHRQ], 2009).

The microsystems linkage to patient safety occurs at various levels with the patient as the focus of all care provided. This linkage means that the leadership sets the vision and purpose, provides a supportive environment, and allocates resources for patient safety. Leadership develops goals and aligns the various microsystems with those goals.

Continuous education and training is based on patient safety concepts and application of quality tools. Staff must also learn how to effectively communicate with each other and with their patients.

Effective communication stems from staff trusting each other to communicate honestly and with self-respect and respect for the other person. Continuous process improvement occurs on a daily basis as the team cares for patients and learns from errors made.

Fractal Organizations

Health care is still provided by tiered, multilayer organizations, in which lines of authority report according to various categories of services. There is more emphasis on task goals than on social goals. As a

FIGURE 7.1
An example of a fractal: Each branch is a graphic iteration
of the preceding pattern.

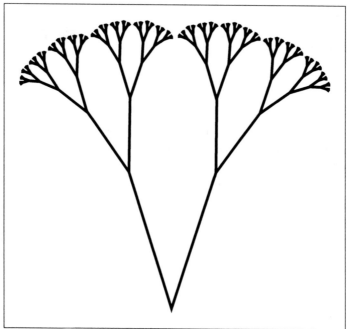

Printed with permission from J. Myers

result of this organizational design, numerous silos of management have been created. Communication across these silos is fragmented and information flow is dysfunctional.

A fractal organization, according to StrateGems Smart Situations (2010), is an organizational model for a cooperative workplace that is based on nature's patterns. There is a constant flow and exchange of information that enables the organization to quickly adapt to changing environments and evolve in an organic fashion.

Fractal organizations have identifiable characteristics. The culture of leadership and shared vision permeate throughout the organization to produce self-organizing units that drive both the change process and the innovation. The shared purpose fully utilizes collective intelligence, and the leaders are the conduits of information and resource flow. Patterns in nature (see Figure 7.1), such as honeycombs in beehives and geese flying in organized "V" arrangements, are compared to organizations' structures and communication patterns. The hierarchical organizational chart is not conducive to responding rapidly to changing environmental demands. Fractal organizations stay focused on the aims of the system (StrateGems, 2010). Fractals are replicable units that are similar to micro-systems, which are also replicable units of groups with purpose, struc-tures, processes, and goals. Fractals are patterns that exist at the micro level that shape the patterns of behavior that exist at the macro level.

The Baldrige Model

The Baldrige model (see Figure 7.2) provides a conceptual framework in which to build health care systems that strive continually for excellence. The Baldrige principles become embedded in the daily operations on a daily basis.

Since 1988, U.S. organizations have competed to win the Malcolm Baldrige National Quality Award, which is the nation's premier award for performance excellence and quality achievement.

This award program was established by Congress in 1987 to raise awareness about the use of quality and performance excellence as a competitive edge in a business strategy. Later, in 1999, health care and

FIGURE 7.2

Baldrige Model. (Springer thanks the Baldrige National Quality Program at the National Institute of Standards and Technology for the use of the Baldrige Model from the criteria for performance excellence.)

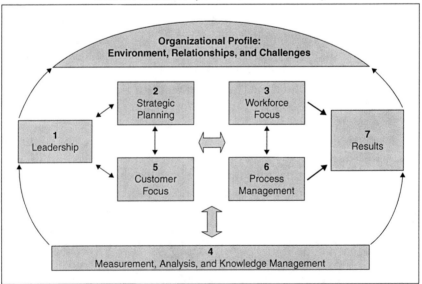

education were added to the award program (National Institute of Standards and Technology [NIST], 2010).

The Baldrige model is a systems model that is consistent with the aims of the Joint Commission and the IOM's report *To Err Is Human: Building a Safer Health System* (2000).

The Baldrige model has seven categories (see Figure 7.2): leadership; strategic planning; focus on patient, other customers, and markets; measurement, analysis, and knowledge management; staff focus; process management; and organizational performance results.

Leadership: Examines how the senior leadership addresses organizational values, guides the governance system, and establishes performance expectations. This includes how the leadership addresses its ongoing responsibilities to the public and how the leadership practices good citizenship.

Strategic planning: Examines how an organization goes about establishing its strategic objectives, taking into account its competitive position in the marketplace. This includes deployment of goals, objectives, action plans, and monitoring and assessing progress toward goals.

Focus on patients, other customers, and markets: Examines how the organization goes about determining the requirements, expectations, and the preferences of its patients, other customers, and markets. This includes how the organization builds ongoing, sustainable relationships with customers.

Measurement, analysis, and knowledge management: Examines how the organization handles analysis and management of data, including the transformation of data to information that is useful, reliable, and valid. This area is the performance management system.

Staff focus: Examines how the organization manages its human capital, which is the most valuable capital. Also, it deals with alignment of staff toward achieving organizational goals.

Process management: Examines how the organization identifies, manages, and improves its key processes that deliver health care services to patients.

Organizational performance results: Examines how the organization provides evidence of continuous improvement and performance in each of the categories: customer satisfaction, financial and marketplace performance, human resources, supplier and partner performance, operational performance, and governance and social responsibility.

Elements from the Baldrige model are included in all hospital accreditation programs.

ISO 9001:2000

The ISO is also a model for quality and patient safety. It has the capacity to be synergistic with accreditation efforts and to increase reliability of key processes.

The ISO was established in 1946 to promote the development of international standards and related activities such as conformity assessment to facilitate the exchange of goods and services worldwide (ISO, n.d.). ISO is a network of national standards institutes of 160 countries, with one member per country. The U.S. member body is named the ANSI. According to the NIST (2003), the Baldrige Award is very different than the ISO 9000.

The ISO 9000 was published in 1987 by the ISO, in Geneva, Switzerland, with the aim to achieve an efficient quality conformance system.

According to the Innovative Quality Solutions Company (2006), ISO 9001:2000 certification promotes the adoption of a process approach when developing, implementing, and improving the system's effectiveness of its quality management system. Departments such as Blood Banks and Laboratory have been certified by ISO for many years. The ISO 9000 enables the health care organization to break down silos with use of the quality management system as the driver for conformance to established requirements. The primary aim is to meet customer requirements.

The focus of the Baldrige model is to build a results-oriented system that aims to excel. ISO complements the Baldrige model by increasing the reliability of the quality management system by developing its own internal auditing system.

CONCLUSIONS

Many health care organizations have added layers of complexity without considering the organizational architecture. All elements within a system have the capacity to enhance the work or hinder the work. Patient safety and accreditation require consideration of using new models to achieve the desired outcomes in these areas. At the microsystem level, staff interact on a daily basis with each other, with patients, and with families to produce outcomes, one patient at a time. It makes sense to develop organizational structures in support of the microsystems and in alignment with system aims. Optimization of the system requires continuous study and adaptation of the sometimes competing and conflicting ongoing interactions of the subsystems. The use of models is essential for alignment of the various elements when the achievement of patient safety and accreditation is viewed as a journey toward being an HRO.

REFERENCES

Agency for Healthcare Research and Quality. (2009). *Clinical microsystems tools and resources.* Retrieved January, 20, 2011, from http://www.innovations. ahrq.gov/content.aspx?id=2468

American Association of Colleges of Nursing. (2006). *Hallmarks of quality and patient safety: Recommended baccalaureate competencies and curricular guidelines to assure high quality and safe patient care.* Retrieved May 21, 2010, from http://www.aacn.nche.edu/publications/pdf/ Qual&PatientSafety.pdf

Benner, P., Sutphen, M., Leonard, V., & Day, L., (2009). *Educating nurses: A call for radical transformation.* Retrieved May 20, 2010, from http://www .carnegiefoundation.org/elibrary/educating-nurses-highlights

Bromley, M., & Franklin, A. (2007). Bromely, M., & Franklin, A. *Joint Commission to extend time to antibiotic administration.* Retrieved May 20, 2010, from http://www.acep.org/content.aspx?id=30132

Graves, N. (2004). *Economics and preventing hospital-acquired infection.* Retrieved May 21, 2010, from http://www.cdc.gov/ncidod/eid/vol10no4/ 02-0754.htm

Huber, D. L. (2000). *Leadership and nursing care management* (3rd ed.). Philadelphia, PA: Saunders Elsevier.

Innovative Quality Solutions Company. (2006). *Differences and similarities between the Malcolm Baldrige Award* (Ohio Partnership for Excellence Award) and the ISO 9001:2000. Standard Retrieved May 20, 2010, from http://www .iqsconsulting.net/resources/Differences_and_Similarities_Between_ the_Baldrige_Award_and_ISO_9000_Standard.pdf

Institute for Healthcare Improvement. (n.d.). *Guidelines for using patient stories with Boards of Directors.* Retrieved January 30, 2011, from http://www. ihi.org/IHI/Topics/LeadingSystemImprovement/Leadership/Tools/ GuidelinesforUsingPatientStorieswithBoardsofDirectors.htm

International Organization for Standardization. (n.d.). *About ISO.* Retrieved January 30, 2011, from http://www.iso.org/iso/about.htm

Jennings, B. M., Disch, J., & Senn, L. (2008). Chapter 20. Leadership. In R. G. Hughes (Ed.), *Patient safety and quality: An evidence-based handbook for nurses.* Retrieved August 1, 2010, from http://www.ahrq.gov/qual/ nurseshdbk/

Joint Commission. (2009). *Hospital accreditation standards.* Oakbrook Terrace, IL: Joint Commission on Accreditation of Healthcare Organizations.

Joint Commission. (2011). *Standard MS.01.01.01: Hospital and critical access hospital accreditation program.* Retrieved January 30, 2011, from http://www .jointcommission.org/standard_ms010101/

Kane, R. L., Shamliyan, T., Mueller, C., Duval, S., & Wilt, T. J. (2007). *Nurse staffing and quality of patient care.* Evidence report/technology assessment No. 151. Prepared by the Minnesota Evidence Based Practice Center under Contract No 290-02-0009. ARHQ Publication No. 07-E005.

Kohn, L. T., Corrigan, J. M., & Donaldson, M. S. (Eds.). (2000). *To err is human: Building a safer health system.* Washington, DC: Doubleday.

Mello, M. M., Studdert, D. M., & Thomas, E. J. (2008). *Who pays for medical errors? An Analysis of adverse event costs, the medical liability system, and incentives for patient safety improvement?* Retrieved May 21, 2010, from http://www.commonwealthfund.org/Content/Publications/In-the-Literature/2008/Apr/Who-Pays-for-Medical-Errors---An-Analysis-of-Adverse-Event-Costs--the-Medical-Liability-System--and.aspx

Mohr, J. J., Batalden, P., & Barach, P. (2004). *Integrating patient safety into clinical microsystem.* Retrieved May 21, from http://rds.epi-ucsf.org/ticr/syllabus/courses/66/2009/10/08/Lecture/readings/microsystem_ref.pdf

Nadler, D. A., Gerstein, M., S., Shaw, R. B., (1992). *Organizational architecture: Designs for changing organizations.* San Francisco: Josssey-Bass.

Nadler, D. A., Tushman, M. L., & Nadler, M. (1997). *Competing by design: The power of organizational architecture.* New York: Oxford University Press.

National Institute of Standards and Technology (2003). *Frequently asked questions about the Malcolm Baldrige National Quality Award.* Retrieved 21 May, 2010, from http://www.nist.gov/public_affairs/factsheet/baldfaqs.cfm

National Institute of Standards and Technology (2010). *History.* Cheltenham, UK: Nelson Thomas Ltd. Retrieved May 20, 2010.

National Patient Safety Foundation (2010). *Unmet needs: Teaching physicians to provide safe patient care.* Lucian Leape Institute Roundtable on Reforming Medical Education. Retrieved January 25, 2011, from http://www.npsf.org/pr/pressrel/2010-03-10.php

Parsley, K., & Corrigan, P. (1999). *Quality improvement in healthcare* (2nd ed).

Provonost, P. (2010). *Death rates not best judge of hospital quality, researchers say.* Retrieved May 20, 2010, from http://www.hopkinsmedicine.org/Press_releases/2010/04_21b_10.html

Reid, P. P., Compton, W. D., Grossman, J. H., & Fanjiang, G. (Eds.). (2005). *Building a better delivery system: A new engineering/healthcare partnership.* Washington, DC: National Academies Press.

Robinson, C. (n.d.). *Chapter 5: Nursing care delivery systems.* Retrieved January 11, 2011, http://www.bookdev.com/pearson/osborn/dap/chapters/m05_osbo 1023_01_se_c05.pdf

Rouse, W. B. (2008). *Health care as a complex adaptive system: Implications for design and management.* Retrieved May 20, 2010, from http://www.nae .edu/Publications/TheBridge/Archives/EngineeringandtheHealthCare DeliverySystem/HealthCareasaComplexAdaptiveSystemImplications forDesignandManagement.aspx

Schyve, P. M. (2005). *Systems thinking and patient safety.* Retrieved, May, 20, 2010, from http://www.ncbi.nlm.nih.gov/bookshelf/br.fcgi?book=aps 2&part=A5987

Senge, P. M. (1990). *The fifth discipline: The art and practice of the learning organization.* New York: Doubleday.

StrateGems. (2010). *Transformational architecture.* Retrieved May 22, 2010, from http://www.strategems.com/fractalorgcharts.htm

III

*The Myers Model for Patient
Safety and Accreditation*

8

Overview of the Myers Model for Patient Safety and Accreditation and Its Application in Health Care .

M odels are a way of explaining abstract or complex concepts through a visual reference that makes it easier to apply to the real world. The Myers Model for Patient Safety and Accreditation covers elements that should be used when conducting strategic planning for patient safety and accreditation efforts (see Figure 8.1). The model—based heavily on the work of Senge (1990), Nadler, Gerstein, and Shaw (1992), Wheatley (1999), and Nelson et al. (2002)—involves three levels: system level, unit level (microsystem), and individual level. At the systems level is leadership, which determines the right thing to do. Leadership decisions affect the entire system. At the unit level is the frontline staff who care for patients on a daily basis. How the leadership designs the unit level determines how well work-flow processes are performed. This also determines the level of safety provided to patients. The individual level is where the leadership design resides, which helps to shape the unit level so that the environment can be safe, effective, equitable, timely, efficient, and employee centered. Workers need to be fully engaged in their work and committed and empowered to learn and adapt within a changing environment.

FIGURE 8.1
The Myers Model for Patient Safety and Accreditation.

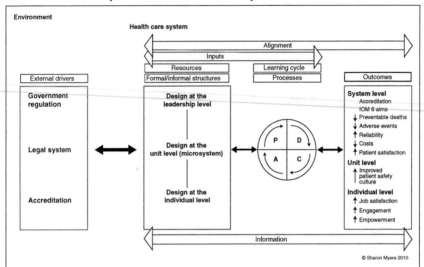

All of these levels continuously exchange information and are influenced by each other. All systems have inputs, throughputs, outputs,
and outcomes.

The Myers Model for Patient Safety and Accreditation (see
Figure 8.1) has several elements within it, and all must be present and
aligned to achieve the aims, or expected outcomes, of the system—at the
system, unit, and individual levels. All of the elements are interrelated
and affect each other on a continual basis. What follows is a general
overview of the elements within the Myers Model for Patient Safety and
Accreditation. Chapters 9, 10, and 11 provide details for key elements
within the model. Chapter 9 presents information for organizational design at the leadership level; Chapter 10 discusses organizational design
at the unit (microsystems) level; and Chapter 11 provides information for
organizational design at the individual level.

ENVIRONMENT

All health care systems are influenced by their environment, and the environment is influenced by the health care system as well. The environment includes, but is not limited to, regulatory and legal requirements,

reimbursement requirements, market requirements, political and economic requirements, advancing technologic requirements, and the effects of the environmental forces on the population and local community served. Health care systems are open, complex systems; they continually adapt or become extinct. For example, if a hospital did well in performance measures but did not manage their finances well, then that hospital may either be sold to a larger health care group or close. Technologic advances are another area that increasingly require a health care organization to decide on the risks involved in being one of the first to implement the new technology or to adopt a wait-and-see attitude and then being perhaps one of the last to implement the new technology. Here, each decision has inherent organizational risks and benefits.

ACCREDITATION

Accreditation, as an element in the external environment, drives patient safety and quality agendas through a set of dynamic standards that require compliance by a health care organization. When the health care organization utilizes robust quality tools to increase reliability of compliance to standards that are evidence based, then there is an increased likelihood of providing safer care in that particular process.

The WHO in 2008 published a paper developed by an expert panel on health systems development; health technology and patient safety which described accreditation as an external review of quality that comprises four primary components:

1. Accreditation is based on a set of written and published standards.
2. The reviews are conducted by professional peers.
3. The accreditation process is an external review, meaning that the process is carried out by an independent agency.
4. The aim of accreditation is to encourage organizational development.

National accrediting bodies require sufficient autonomy, human capacity, and the financial resources to be sustainable and to operate effectively.

Many private insurers in the United States require accreditation as a prerequisite for reimbursement. At the same time, all accredited organizations must comply with the CMS COPs to obtain federal reimbursement for Medicare or Medicaid programs. Increasingly, accreditation has the potential to be the key external driver for implementing effective quality and patient safety programs. And accreditation programs are increasingly adding patient safety processes to their standards.

ALIGNMENT

Alignment means having an arrangement that is in a straight line or in parallel lines. Alignment is an essential element of the Myers model. When geese fly in the sky, they fly in a perfect V formation. If one bird drops out of the formation, another bird is right there to take its place (see Figure 8.2).

Another example of alignment is music played in harmony. When you hear such music, you can immediately sense the alignment of the various instruments. Each musician knows his or her role and produces the exact sound that aligns in harmony with how the other musicians are playing.

FIGURE 8.2

Example of alignment: Geese flying in formation.

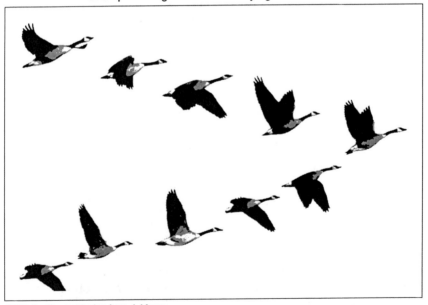

Printed with permission from J. Myers

Similarly, all of the organizational elements at each level—leadership, unit, and individual—must be aligned to achieve potential system optimization. Alignment ensures that everyone in the organization is working together to achieve the aims of the system. Alignment also occurs through use of formal and informal means. There is vertical communication through the management hierarchy downward to the department level and then the staff level. Horizontal alignment is enhanced through numerous project interdisciplinary teams and through designing the work environment in a manner that shapes desired culture and behaviors.

If one of the elements is dysfunctional, however, then all of the other elements are affected. For example, if the leadership team does not work well together, this dysfunctional social interaction affects the organizational culture, which can also have an impact on patient safety and the culture of patient safety in the organization.

Another example of the importance of alignment relates to human resource policies. If the health care organization has a cohesive leadership but the human resource policies are rigid, and do not allow for attracting and retaining the best candidates, then the system suffers dysfunction at all levels. Human resource policies structure the design of human capital. If the right staff are not selected for the work assigned to them, then the system may not have the capacity to be optimized.

RESOURCES

The amount of resources that a health care organization has determines the types of strategies from which they can choose. Limited financial resources limit health care organizations' abilities to purchase and adopt new technologies.

Resources are the fuel that drives the train, and all health care systems are feeling the crunch of decreasing finances.

The Robert Wood Johnson Foundation (RWJF) reported in 2001 that hospital beds decreased by nearly 28 percent between 1980 and 1997. More efficient hospitals were not necessarily the type most likely to survive. More financially secure hospitals with greater financial resources relative to patient volume were more likely to remain open than their efficient counterparts. Survival of the fattest instead of the fittest prevailed.

The American Hospital Association (AHA) (2010) reported that hospitals are continuing to feel the lingering effects of the economic recession. Seventy percent of hospitals reported decreased volumes of elective procedures. There have also been significant enrollment increases in Medicaid, Children's Health Insurance Program (CHIP), and/or other programs for low-income populations. These government programs tend to underpay hospitals, which places an additional strain on the hospital's financial resources. Forty-four percent of hospitals surveyed reported reduced access to capital. According to AHA, this reduced access to capital comes at a time when hospitals are trying to implement electronic health records and qualify as "meaningful users" to receive financial incentives contained in the American Recovery and Reinvestment Act (ARRA) and avoid future penalties.

Hospitals that have more resources have a greater likelihood to implement capital investments for patient safety. These hospitals also have greater choices for strategy selection in terms of staffing, equipment, space, and acquisitions.

Staffing resources, of course, are critical for patient safety efforts— and the number of states that mandate controversial nurse/patient ratios (guaranteed number of patients that each nurse can be assigned) are increasing.

Downsizing, restructuring, and/or reengineering, especially when implemented without considering their impact on individual staff members, may not yield the financial outcomes intended.

A review of the literature by Gandolfi (2008) in this regard noted that only a few firms reported some financial improvements; however, the majority of firms that were surveyed were unable to report improved levels of productivity, efficiency, effectiveness, and profitability. Gandolfi also stated that there have been social consequences to downsizing as well. The staff who remain behind become resentful at having to do more work for the same pay as they continue to work for a company they no longer trust.

In 1996, Mick and Wise reported results from a national sample of 797 rural hospitals from 1983 to 1988. The results indicated that although approximately 15 percent of all rural hospitals had experienced downsizing, a positive association between downsizing and financial performance was unconfirmed.

Appelbaum, Lavigne-Schmidt, Peytchev, and Shapiro (1999) performed a five-year review of the literature on the management practice of downsizing and its related costs from 1994 to 1998. This information was used to analyze the positive and negative effects of downsizing. They concluded that, even though there could be many positive outcomes to a downsizing project, in the end, the negative outcomes outweighed the positive.

Before health care organizations decide to downsize as a reduced cost strategy, careful consideration of the risks versus the benefits needs to be performed. Downsizing also needs to be done within an ethical framework.

FORMAL STRUCTURES AND PROCESSES

Formal organizational structures such as the organizational chart, committee design, work group assignments, degree of centralization versus decentralization, rules and regulations, specific organizational policies and procedures, and arrangements of the work environment set boundaries for expected behavioral norms. Formal structure is the blueprint on which organizational activities are built and are high in technical/task orientation. According to Senge (2004), "we create the structure and then the structure creates us." Patient safety requires formal structures to be in alignment with patient safety and quality concepts.

INFORMAL ORGANIZATIONAL STRUCTURES AND PROCESSES

Informal organizational structures are high in social interactions and communication networks. Informal leaders emerge by virtue of their social skills, knowledge skills, and/or proximity to formal power positions. Wheatley (1999) posited that leadership's role was to create a strong vision based on mutual, shared values and allow for self-organizing systems to emerge. Relationships within the system are essential for the leadership to actively engage in the culture to provide meaning and logic.

ORGANIZATIONAL CULTURE: AN INFORMAL STRUCTURE

Schein (1984) defined organizational culture as the pattern of "basic assumptions that a given group has invented, discovered, or developed in learning to cope with its problems of external adaptation and internal integration, and that have worked well enough to be considered valid, and, therefore, to be taught to new members as the correct way to perceive, think, and feel in relation to those problems."

According to Schein, there are three levels in the organizational culture:

1. The first level is what is called "visible artifacts." For example, you can see the size of the offices, the accepted staff attire in the workplace, and how employees greet one another.
2. The second level is at the "value" level. This level helps to explain why staff behave in the manner that they do.
3. The third level is the "underlying assumptions." These assumptions are ingrained into the value system. Schein states that they are typically unconscious and actually determine how the group members perceive information and think and feel about it. These assumptions are so ingrained that they are not debatable because they are accepted by the group as truth.

According to the Agency for Health Care Research and Quality (AHRQ) (n.d.), improvement of the patient safety culture in health care organizations is an essential component for providing safer care to patients.

The Myers model emphasizes the patient safety culture at all levels of the organization (see Figure 8.3).

FIGURE 8.3
Organizational design levels.

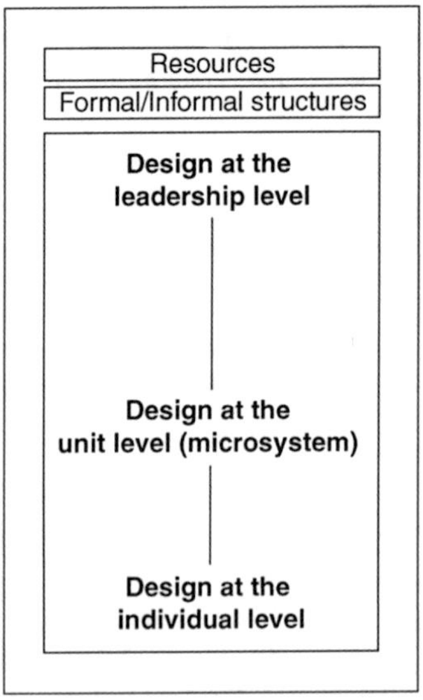

Resources

Formal/Informal structures

**Design at the
leadership level**

**Design at the
unit level (microsystem)**

**Design at the
individual level**

LEADERSHIP DESIGN AT THE SYSTEM LEVEL

Leadership design at the system level plays a central role in the Myers Model for Patient Safety and Accreditation. The model reviews the essential roles of leadership vision, purpose, ethics, values, reward and recognition systems, and role modeling to positively influence the patient safety culture and outcomes. Examples of the types of organizational formal structures are discussed in more detail. More generally, leadership design must be supportive to the microsystems level and to the individual level. The leadership decides the right thing to do and must be accountable for patient safety within their organization.

Nursing leadership is part of the leadership team. As such, nurse executives must have equal voices in the board room when decision making is done. It is essential that the leadership group works within a team structure.

MICROSYSTEMS DESIGN AT THE UNIT LEVEL

Microsystems design at the unit level has the capacity for making the largest impact on patient safety and quality. Microsystems are a small group of people working together on a daily basis to provide care to a defined population. This unit performs key processes and produces measureable outcomes. These groups are also supported by business and a shared information environment (Nelson et al., 2002). Microsystems are located at the interface between the provider group and the patient and family. Because adverse events occur at this interface of care, it is essential to build effective microsystems.

Nelson describes nine success characteristics associated with high performance: leadership, culture, organizational support, patient focus, staff focus, interdependence of the care team, information, information technology (IT), and process improvement. Microsystems have characteristics of self-directed work teams that have defined goals, membership, and leadership support for building the support systems and communication flow that is necessary for effective work flow. Many of these concepts are congruent with principles contained within the Baldrige model and are explored in detail in later chapters.

DESIGN AT THE INDIVIDUAL LEVEL

The design at the individual level needs to mirror the six aims of the system, as stated by the IOM: to be safe, effective, timely, efficient, equitable, and patient centered. For the staff to deliver patient-centered care, the system needs to be employee centered.

Human capital is the most valuable asset of any organization. Weatherly (2003) defines human capital as the collective sum of all of the attributes, life experience, knowledge, creativity, energy, and enthusiasm that staff choose to invest in their work.

Deming's *Out of Crisis* (1982) emphasized the importance of continuous training to improve skills, improve flexibility in job assignments, and gain competitive advantage. Training needs to occur at all levels within the organization. All employees need to appreciate variation and its effects on processes.

Deming also coined the phrase "drive out fear." He believed that employees could not perform their best when they were afraid of losing their jobs.

Patient safety is one area in which staff members cannot be afraid of punishment when they do the right thing and report honest mistakes. The work environment needs to be created in a manner that increases the likelihood that staff will not make a mistake. For example, hand hygiene compliance is difficult to sustain. If the hospital used technology to integrate hand hygiene into the work-flow process making it mandatory for the staff to wash their hands prior to touching a patient, then compliance would be built into the work-flow process instead of relying on inspection.

Poor communication and team interactions also contribute to medical errors. A Harvard study in 2002 reported that negative team factors in the operating room environment contributed to delays in 40 percent of all cases studied and were responsible for 30 percent of adverse events (Controlled Risk Insurance Company or Risk Management Foundation [CRICO or RMF], n.d.).

Many times, hospitals implement teams and then wonder why the teams did not perform as expected. Patient safety demands the use of effective teamwork; poor communication is frequently a contributing cause for adverse events. There needs to be a greater emphasis on building team competencies at the unit level.

Baker, Gustafason, Beaubien, Salas, and Barach (2005) defined a team as having five key characteristics:

1. The team is made up of two or more individuals.
2. The team members have specific roles, they perform specific tasks, and they interact or coordinate to achieve a common goal or outcome.

3. The team makes decisions.

4. The team has specialized knowledge and skills, often functioning under conditions of high workload.

5. The team differs from small groups in which teams personify a collective action that is the result of task interdependency. Team members make adjustments to one another, either sequentially or at the same time, in an effort to accomplish assigned goals.

Team member competencies are the knowledge, skills, and attitudes that each team member has for successfully accomplishing the work of the team. According to Baker et al. (2005), primary teamwork competencies exist within each domain of knowledge, skills, and attitudes. For example, under the competency of knowledge, each team member needs to have a shared understanding of what the goals or objectives are, as well as the resources available to achieve the goals or objectives. The knowledge of the team members must also adapt to any changes that occur.

An example of skill required is that there has to be mutual performance monitoring to ensure that the project is proceeding as expected and that the correct actions have been followed.

An example of attitude competencies is the positive attitude that team members possess and the general mood or climate of the team's interactions with each other. It is important to note that just implementing team structures does not automatically result in effective teamwork. Team members need to have the right knowledge, skills, and attitudes along with adequate organizational resources and support. Team training, with the use of scenario-based training (SBT) or event-based approach techniques (EBAT), has shown promise as a strategy for training care providers who must coordinate their efforts in high-risk areas, such as intensive care units and emergency room departments.

The complexity of health care demands a new way of doing the work; otherwise, different results will not be achieved. Communication is frequently cited as one contributing cause for adverse events, and working in teams who have clear goals and objectives for the day's work may assist with improving the quality of communication between the various disciplines. Individual competency in team participation is essential to building a safer work environment for patient care.

According to AHRQ (n.d.), safe health care depends on highly trained individuals who have very different roles and responsibilities, acting together in the best interests of the patient. Communication barriers and poor teamwork can lead to clinical adverse events. Specific teamwork training in health care includes Team STEPPS (Team Strategies and Tools to Enhance Performance and Patient Safety). This program was developed by the U.S. Department of Defense and the AHRQ . The Team STEPPS training material is free online. Other free sources for team training include the following.

The WHO has a WHO Patient Safety Curriculum for Medical Schools available for download free of charge at www.who.int/patientsafety/education/curriculum/download/en/index.html.

The University of Michigan Health System (UMHS) Patient Safety Toolkit is available at www.med.umich.edu/patientsafetytoolkit/curriculum.htm.

The Massachusetts Medical Society (MMS) Patient Safety Curriculum is available at www.massmed.org/AM/Template.cfm?Section=Home6&CONTENTID=3925&TEMPLATE=/CM/HTMLDisplay.cfm.

The Washington State Medical Association (WSMA) Patient Safety Curriculum is available at www.wsma.org/medical_professionalism/patient-safety-curriculum.cfm.

The Curriculum for Patient Safety from the Society of Academic Emergency Medicine (SAEM) is available at www.saem .org/SAEMDNN/Portals/0/IGroups/Patient/2006June6/patient_safety.pd.

PROCESSES

Processes are a series of interrelated tasks that produce a result, which leads to outputs and outcomes. Every department within a health care organization has key processes in which they must perform their role to successfully achieve a desired goal.

Many nursing processes have great opportunities for improvement at the unit level. Hendrick, Chow, Skierczynski, and Zhenqiang (2008) performed time-and-motion studies to document how nurses actually spend their time. A total of 767 nurses participated. Documentation accounted for 35.3 percent (147.5 minutes per day); medication administration, 17.2 percent (72 minutes per day); and care coordination 20.6 percent (86 minutes day). Actual nursing practice time for patient assessment and reading of vital signs was only 7.2 percent (31 minutes) of nursing time. The remaining 19.7 percent of nurses' time (82.5 minutes per day) was shown as "other." Nurses at the unit level have great opportunities to structure and integrate their roles within a multidisciplinary team environment.

PERFORMANCE MEASURES FOR CRITICAL PROCESSES

Patterns of performance are part of the information required at the unit (or microsystem) level to benchmark information and continually improve performance.

Performance measurement, according to the Council of Medical Specialty Societies (2007), requires a measurement system that is purposeful, comprehensive, and transparent. The organizations described in this section all have various methods for measuring performance.

Major stakeholders within the government are the CMS, the AHRQ, the Medicare Payment Advisory Commission (MedPAC), the U.S. Government Accountability Office (GAO), state Medicaid agencies, and state programs, all of which publicly report health quality data.

The NQF, the Joint Commission, and the National Committee for Quality Assurance (NCQA) are considered public–private partnerships.

Collaborations and alliances include the Assessment and Qualifications Alliance (AQA), the Hospital Quality Alliance (HQA), the Quality Alliance Steering Committee (QASC), the Physician's Consortium for Performance Improvement (PCPI), and the Leapfrog Group.

Performance measure is an essential component of process improvement and patient safety efforts.

The National Healthcare Quality Report published by AHRQ (2010) is developed from more than 200 measures across four dimensions of quality: patient safety, timeliness, effectiveness, and patient centeredness. Some outcome measures got worse instead of improving from the previous year. In adult surgery patients with postoperative catheter-associated urinary tract infection outcomes got worse by 3.6 percent, and in those with postoperative sepsis, it got worse by 8 percent. It was felt that this worsening might be due to increased detectability of HAIs. There were also significant differences between individuals with private insurance versus no insurance related to preventive services and diabetes management.

The real challenge is separating the trivial many from the critical few that will impact the IOM's six specific system aims the most.

Just because something can be measured does not necessarily mean it should be measured. Measurements need to occur at critical phases of the continuum of care, from keeping people healthy to providing palliative care at the end-of-life. These measurements require a cohesive, integrated approach with consensus from all stakeholders, and include the patient's perspectives as stakeholder as well.

LEARNING CYCLE

Shewart started the learning cycle of specification, production, and inspection that was modified by Deming in 1950 and later applied in Japan as the plan-do-check-act- (PDCA) cycle (Moen & Norman, n.d.).

Since that time, many modifications of the basic PDCA model have been implemented; yet all involve having a vision, a shared purpose, concrete aims, a team that maps out the current process, and pilot projects that engage recommended changes to test capacities for improvement. Use of teams enables staff to see beyond their own departments and acquire new skills related to functioning effectively within a team framework to get work accomplished.

IHI (n.d.) emphasizes three fundamental questions that must be answered in any order:

What are we trying to accomplish? The team must have aims that have time lines and are measureable. The population that is affected needs to be defined.

How will we know that the change our team makes is an improvement? The only way the team will know if change is an improvement is to collect data. The measurements selected by the team need to be consistent with the aims and provide the team with enough information to know if they are progressing, getting worse, or staying the same.

What changes can we make that will result in an improvement? The team must identify the changes that will most likely result in an improvement.

Plan-Do-Study-Act (PDSA) cycle: The team goes through the learning cycle in which changes are tested, the results are shared, and the team acts on what is learned.

Implementing changes: After the team's pilot on a small scale is evaluated as successful through the use of several PDSA cycles, the change can be attempted on a larger scale.

Spreading changes: After success at the unit level, the team can spread the changes to other areas within the organization.

According to Peter Senge (1990), a learning organization is one in which "people continually expand their capacity to create the results they truly desire, where new and expansive patterns of thinking are nurtured, where collective aspiration is set free and where people are continually learning to learn together." This involves a hierarchy consisting of four levels according to Trivedi (n.d.).

Level one: Staff learn facts, knowledge, processes, and procedures. In hospitals, staff do this within their own functional areas of responsibility. Think of learning how to play a piano; basic skills of learning how to play basic notes are repeated over and over again. A new team coming together for the first time needs to learn how to communicate with each other effectively by practicing basic skills over and over again.

Level two: Staff learn new job skills that are transferable to other situations. An example of this would be learning team skills. In learning how to play a piano, transferability applies to being able to play new songs with the same notes.

Level three: Staff learn to adapt. They apply team skills at the unit level where the PDCA cycle is ongoing, one day at a time, one patient at a time. This is analogous to playing new songs on the piano with variation of the beats.

Level four: Staff learn to learn. This is the breakthrough level. As staff learn to learn through the use of teams, innovation and creativity occur instead of just adaptation. This is analogous to composing new songs at every opportunity instead of just playing the songs already known.

The above levels occur at the individual level, the unit level, and the organizational level (see Figure 8.4).

FIGURE 8.4
Outcomes.

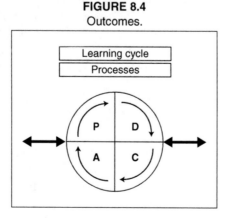

OUTCOMES

System Level

Health care should be safe, effective, timely, efficient, equitable, and patient centered. There should be a decrease in preventable deaths and other adverse events. There should be increased reliability of processes and reduced costs as non-value-added steps are eliminated. When the design of the microsystems is effective, there should be higher patient satisfaction with care. Accreditation as a successful outcome measure is also increasingly an aim of the health care system.

Unit Level (Micro System)

The patient safety culture is improved. There is an increase in the team's authority to make decisions for patients and improvement of processes. There will be new models for nursing care delivery that build on inter-disciplinary teamwork with nursing taking the lead for coordination and integration of the care provided to patients on a daily basis.

Individual Level

When the environment at the unit level is shaped in a manner that en-hances the ability for employees to be safe, effective, timely, efficient, eq-uitable, and employee centered, staff can ensure that the IOM's six aims are achieved, one patient at a time. Staff are empowered to make deci-sions at the unit level, and nurses at the unit level self-govern their areas with boundaries to set the leadership tone. There are self-directed inter-disciplinary teams at the unit level that communicate patient goals on a daily basis and then measure to see if, at the end of day, the goals were achieved. When goals are not met, the team makes adaptations. This re-sults in increased job satisfaction and increased engagement of staff.

INFORMATION

Information is the foundation of the patient safety model. IT is criti-cal to implement effective quality and patient safety programs. IT is increasingly used, not just at the system level but also at the provider level. Medical information is available to health care professionals where and when needed. The amount of information required for effective medical decision making cannot be stored by memory in a person's brain anymore; it is just too much information that constantly changes.

Implementation of information systems requires strategic planning with involvement of key stakeholders for success. Computerized physician order entry (CPOE), depending on how it its implemented, can have unintended consequences. Ash, Sittig, Campbell, Guappone, and Dykstra (2006) reported that CPOE can create shifts in power, control, and autonomy. They recommend heavy clinician involvement in planning for CPOE.

The health care organization cannot survive without having a robust information system. Health care is becoming increasingly complex. Information systems have the potential to integrate clinical, financial, and administrative processes and also drive decision making at the system level, the unit level (microsystem), and the individual level. It is the foundation for effective quality and patient safety efforts.

Information should be provided as close to real-time as can be achieved at the unit level. Data display yields information on which decisions can be made at the unit level and at the system level. Having access to real-time information increases feedback, learning, and improvement.

Real-time data at the unit level has the potential to drive decision making at the place where it belongs: at the patient's bedside.

Electronic medical records have U.S. government stimulus funds for their implementation, and providers who do not implement an IT system by 2015 will see shrinking Medicare payments. Bennett (2009) reported that even with incentives, "70 percent of hospitals still have a long journey." He reported that large, urban hospitals are more likely to have health informatics systems than smaller more rural hospitals. This is because the large, urban hospitals are more likely to have more resources to invest in capital purchases such as IT and can also absorb the continued high maintenance costs better than the smaller, more rural hospitals.

HOW TO USE THE MYERS MODEL FOR PATIENT SAFETY AND ACCREDITATION

Health care systems are not safe. They are not safe for patients and they are not safe for the workers who provide care for patients. Health care organizations need to build high-reliable organizations. To accomplish this, there needs to be radical change of the health care systems.

Patients need to be able to trust that health care providers will do the right thing, the right way, on time, every time.

Staff working in health care need to be able to trust that the leadership will provide a safe working environment, in which they can provide care.

Every other day that the health care organization continues with the same faulty system design that has harmed patients is one day too long to wait for meaningful change. Every day that the staff experience preventable harm from events such as needle sticks, back injuries from poor ergonomics, and violence that occurs in the workplace is one day too long to wait for meaningful change.

Use of the Myers Model for Patient Safety and Accreditation when developing and implementing patient safety efforts will ensure that the leadership has current, evidence-based information to use in modifying their organizational architecture in a manner that is congruent with their vision, mission, organizational values, and resources. The Myers Model for Patient Safety and Accreditation should be used for key decision making related to the elements within the model, such as degree of centralization versus decentralization, degree of empowerment of teams, culture, and values. Further, the leadership should start with system design at the top and develop effective leadership structures/processes that are congruent with the unit level (microsystems) design.

The mission for health care relates to implementation and sustaining the IOM's six aims: safe, effective, timely, efficient, equitable, and patient centered.

Feedback centered on measurement of outcomes relating to the six aims is essential for organizational learning and improvement. The use of the learning cycle of PDCA along with the measurement of outcomes enables the organization to know the degree of effectiveness of their patient safety and accreditation program.

Safety is a basic minimum aim for a health care organization to achieve and is an ethical imperative. Leaders must transform the current organizational cultures and structures that are preventing change. This is not an easy task because staff within the various groups have wide variation in their cultures and their view of the world.

It is the best interests of the patient that must be the common ground for dialog between diverse groups of staff. Hospital leaders need to provide a clear vision and provide clear boundaries for acceptable behavior expected of their staff. The leadership needs to make it clear that patient safety is the priority. This means putting the patient first with no exceptions.

Leaders also need to recognize that having an engaged workforce will help to create a new health care system where both patients and workers have a high degree of trust in the leaders to do the right thing for patients and for staff.

HOW THE MODEL ASSISTS WITH ACCREDITATION AND PATIENT SAFETY EFFORTS

Accreditation is increasingly being viewed in the global marketplace as a means to implement quality and patient safety in hospitals. Shaw (2003) identified 36 national accreditation programs that were cited in a global study for the WHO. The common areas of emphasis for developed countries included the evaluation of safety, clinical effectiveness, consumer information, development of staff, purchaser intelligence, accountability, and reducing variation.

For developing countries, Shaw stated that the emphasis was on establishment of basic facilities, information, and improving patient access to care. Developing countries may have no established culture of professional responsibility. There may also be very limited resources for staffing, equipment, and building structures related to achieving accreditation.

Within the United States, whole health care networks obtain accreditation for each level of service provided: acute care, ambulatory care, rehabilitation, long-term care, home health care, and so on. Within each phase of care, accreditation standards emphasize staying healthy, and preventive, curative, palliative, and end-of-life care.

Devers, Pham, and Liu (2004) stated that there are three mechanisms for stimulating hospitals to reduce medical errors: professionalism, regulation, and market forces. These authors reported that a quasi-regulatory accrediting body such as the Joint Commission has been the primary driver of hospitals' patient safety initiatives.

The Myers Model for Patient Safety and Accreditation emphasizes accreditation as the one of the key external drivers for patient safety and also as one of expected outcomes. The leaders should compare the various accreditation programs in the United States and determine the one they feel will best assist them to build a safer health care environment.

HOW THE MODEL ASSISTS THE LEADERSHIP'S
DECISION MAKING

The leadership has to decide on how best to select sustainable strategies to achieve patient safety and successful accreditation. Leadership must take an active role in accreditation efforts. This means being available to resolve conflicts, provide resources in a timely fashion where needed, and problem solve with teams when needed. The chapter on leadership design goes into detail about leadership characteristics that will assist in the development of effective clinical microsystems. When hospitals prepare for accreditation, they can use the Myers Model for Patient Safety and Accreditation as a means of building systems with high reliability of their processes that are also compliant with accreditation standards. This high reliability translates into compliance with standards consistently on a daily basis and with safer care provided to patients.

Leadership Resource Decisions

Accreditation costs vary. According to Meldi, Rhoades, and Gippe (2009), the average cost for the Joint Commission services is $33,000 for 3 years, the average cost for Healthcare Facilities Accreditation Program (HFAP) is $25,000 for 3 years, and the average annual cost for Det Norske Veritas (DNV) services is $23,100. Accreditation program costs vary according to the number of surveyors required depending on facility size and complexity. The leadership decides which accreditation system fits their vision, purpose, values, and resources. The leadership may also elect not to use accreditation as an alternative, but rather use the CMS's survey process instead.

Patient safety efforts also require resources invested in IT. According to Newell and Christensen (n.d.), the greatest areas of attention for patient safety have been on CPOE and bar coding medication administration (BCMA) systems. The authors recommend that return on investment metrics include categories related to reduced adverse events, increased satisfaction, and increased staff productivity, with improved work flow.

Leadership Decisions for Structure and Processes

Organizational structures at the system, unit, and individual level need to be congruent to achieve the desired outcomes. The structures that are supportive of accreditation and patient safety efforts include building a patient safety culture, optimizing the use of interdisciplinary teams at the leadership and the unit level, and building patterns of communication that break down silos of information and centralized control.

Structures are developed that enhance communication flow and ensure that the structures, processes, and outcomes required for patient safety and accreditation efforts are developed, implemented, monitored, and continually improved.

Recommended processes to be put in place for patient safety include the NQF's Consensus Standards for Safe Practices. The NQF's mission is "to improve the quality of American healthcare by setting national priorities and goals for performance improvement, endorsing national consensus standards for measuring and publicly reporting on performance, and promoting the attainment of national goals through education and outreach program."

In 2003, the NQF endorsed the first set of Safe Practices (AHRQ, 2003). This set has been continually updated to reflect new evidence. NQF Safe Practices for Better Healthcare update (2010) contains 34 safe practices that include previously endorsed practices and are suited for applicable health care settings across the continuum of care with the aim to reduce the risk of harm to patients resulting from processes, systems, and environments of care.

The 34 safe practices have strong evidence that they are effective in reducing the risk of harm to patients.

You can refer to the *Safe Practices for Better Healthcare: 2010 Update* information in the Appendix A NQF 34 safe practices at the end of this book.

The updated 2010 standards include nursing workforce safe practices with emphasis on nurse staffing plans, and the governing boards' accountability for providing resources that support not only nurse staffing but the ongoing continued learning for increasing knowledge and skills within the work setting. Ongoing competency of direct caregivers is also cited as a safe practice.

Physicians' safe practice for the intensive care units (both adult and pediatric) entails having patients managed only by physicians who have the specific knowledge and skills to care for them. This means physicians should be certified in critical care medicine.

Other examples of 2010 safe practices include, but are not limited to, taking actions to prevent surgical-site infections by implementing evidence-based interventions, taking evidence-based actions to prevent complications associated with ventilator patients, and implementing actions to prevent multidrug-resistant organisms (NQF, 2010).

ACCREDITATION STANDARDS HELP BUILD
PATIENT SAFETY PROCESSES

Another set of processes that should be in place for patient safety are accreditation standards. For example, approximately half of Joint Commission's standards are patient safety related (Joint Commission, 2010).

Joint Commission also publishes Sentinel Event Alerts to stimulate collective learning from SEs reported to them.

Approximately 30 percent of the HFAP's standards are patient safety related. In addition, HFAP endorses the NQF 34 safe practices and includes other patient safety initiatives (HFAP, n.d.)

Finally, DNV supports hospitals to be innovative and supports the initiatives that the hospitals have selected and implemented to guide safe patient-care practices, and DNV holds hospitals accountable to sustain their quality management system (Meldi et al., 2009).

FEEDBACK PROCESS AT THE UNIT AND LEADERSHIP LEVEL

The tracer process consists of using tools that are used to "trace" the care of the patients as they travel through the health care system. Tracers can be designed to focus on key clinical processes such as assessment of patients, provision of care, continuity of care, infection control, and so on. Tracers can also be designed to look at management of key processes such as medication management starting from the supply chain and ending at the patient's bedside with the nurse administering the medication to the patient.

Tracers provide the health care organization an evaluation method to see if processes are operating as they were designed to operate. In other words, if a policy is in writing, are staff implementing the policy as intended?

Aggregate tracers are rich resources of information for the leadership to implement corrective actions where needed.

For example, three of the tracers demonstrated that pain scores above 5 did not have timely intervention. In one instance, the pain score was documented and no actions were taken by the nurse. In two other events, the pain score above 5 remained at 5 after the intervention, and the physician was not notified.

The tracer teams report to the leadership on a regular basis. By integrating tracer teams into the health care organization's structures and processes, a feedback loop is created for the leadership and unit level.

USE OF THE MYERS MODEL BY NURSE EXECUTIVES

Models are a way of explaining complex concepts. The Myers' Model for Patient Safety and Accreditation covers the essential areas that must be considered by the leadership during their strategic planning efforts. Nurse executives should use this model when they are involved in designing clinical microsystems at the unit level or shaping the environment at the individual level. Nurse executives should also use the model to advocate for staff having the right competencies to work in teams. Nurse executives should be involved at strategic planning sessions and be able to offer innovative ideas for work being implemented at the clinical microsystems level.

Nurses at the unit level should use this model to ensure that their multidisciplinary team has the resources and leadership support necessary to provide safe care, one patient at a time. Nurses at the unit level should be able to articulate what information and resources they need to be able to care for patients safely. They should demand that information be as close to real-time as possible so as to let the team evaluate their care on a daily basis.

CONCLUSIONS

The Myers Model for Patient Safety and Accreditation provides a framework for organizational architecture at the systems level, the unit level (microsystem), and the individual level. All of the elements are essential and are interrelated to achieve the six aims of the health care system. Health care should be safe, effective, timely, efficient, equitable, and patient centered. Accreditation is increasingly becoming an external driver for patient safety efforts and when used as an external driver, is an expected outcome of the health care system. When one area of the model is dysfunctional, this adversely affects the entire system. Nurse executives should use the Myers Model for Patient Safety and Accreditation when making strategic choices to develop microsystems and design the environment of nursing practice.

REFERENCES

Agency for Health Care Research and Quality. (2003). *National quality forum finds consensus on 30 patient safety practices.* Retrieved May 29, 2010, from http://www.ahrq.gov/news/press/pr2003/forumpr.htm

Agency for Health Care Research and Quality Publication No 10.0003. (2010). *National healthcare quality report.* Rockville, MD: Agency for Healthcare Research and Quality.

Agency for Health Care Research and Quality. (n.d.). *Patient safety primer: Safety culture.* Retrieved February 1, 2011, from http://psnet.ahrq.gov/primer.aspx?primerID=5

American Hospital Association. (2010). *Hospitals continue to feel lingering effects of the economic recession.* Retrieved May 20, 2010, from http://www.aha.org/aha/research-and-trends/AHA-policy-research/2010.html

Appelbaum, S. H., Lavigne-Schmidt, S., Peytchev. M., & Shapiro, B. (1999). Downsizing: Measuring the costs of failure. *Journal of Management Development, 18*(5), 436–463.

Ash, J. S., Sittig, D. F., Campbell, E., Guappone, K., & Dykstra, R. (2006). *An unintended consequence of CPOE implementation: Shifts in power, control, and autonomy.* AMIA Annual Symposium Proceedings. Retrieved August 1, 2010, from https://www.ncbi.nlm.nih.gov/pmc/articles/PMC1839304/

Baker, D. P., Gustafason, S., Beaubien, J., Salas, E., & Barach, P. (2005). *Medical teamwork and patient safety: Chapter 2. Training teams: The evidence based relation.* Literature review publication No. 05-0053. Agency for Healthcare Research and Quality(AHRQ). http://www.ahrq.gov/qual/medteam/medteam2.htm

Bennett, D. (2009, June 1). Objective measures define EMR adoption levels: Even with incentives, 70% of hospitals still have a long journey. *Managed Healthcare Executive.* Retrieved August 1, 2010 from http://managed-healthcareexecutive.modernmedicine.com/mhe/Technology+Strategy/Objective-measures-define-EMR-adoption-levels/ArticleStandard/Article/detail/601154

Centers for Medicare & Medicaid. (n.d.). *CMS conditions of participation for healthcare.* Retrieved May 23, 2010, from http://www.cms.gov/CFCsAndCoPs

Controlled Risk Insurance Company/Risk Management Foundation (CRICO/RMF). (n.d.). *Communication/teamwork.* Retrieved May 24, 2010, from http://www.rmf.harvard.edu/patient-safety-strategies/communication-teamwork/index.aspx

Council of Medical Specialty Societies: United Health Foundation. (2007). *The measurement of health care performance: A primer from the CMSS.* Retrieved May 22, 2010, from http://www.unitedhealthfoundation.org/

Deming, W. E. (1982). *Out of the crisis*. Cambridge, MA: MIT.

Devers, K. J., Pham, H. H., & Liu, G. (2004). What is driving hospital's patient-safety efforts? *Health Affairs, 23*(2), 103–115.

Gandolfi, F. (2008). Learning from the past--downsizing lessons for managers. *Journal of Management Research, 8*(1), 3–17.

Hendrick, A., Chow, M., Skierczynski, B. A., & Zhenqiang, L. (2008). A 36-hospital time and motion study: How do Medical-Surgical nurses spend their time? *Permanente Journal, 12*(3), 25–34.

Healthcare Facilities Accreditation Program. (n.d.). HFAP: *Healthcare facilities accreditation program: Frequently asked questions*. Retrieved May 29, 2010, from http://www.hfap.org/about/faq.aspx

IHI. (n.d.). *A resource form the institute for healthcare improvement; How to improve; improvement methods*. Retrieved May 25, 2010, http://www.ihi.org/knowledge/Pages/HowtoImprove/default.aspx

Joint Commission. (2010). *Joint commission fact sheets: Facts about patient safety*. Retrieved May 23, 2010, from http://www.jointcommission.org/AboutUs/Fact_Sheets/facts_patient_safety.htm

Meldi, D., Rhoades, F., & Gippe, A. (2009). *The big three: A side-by-side matrix comparing hospital accrediting agencies*. Retrieved May 29, 2010, from http://www.hfap.org/mediacenter/NAMSS%20Synergy%20JanFeb09_Accreditation%20Grid.pdf

Mick, S. S., & Wise, C. G. (1996). Downsizing and financial performance in rural hospitals. *Health Care Management Review, 21*(2), 26–28.

Moen, R., & Norman, C. (n.d.). *Evolution of the PDCA cycle*. Retrieved May 22, 2010, from http://pkpinc.com/files/NA01MoenNormanFullpaper.pdf

Nadler, D. A., Gerstein, M. S., & Shaw, R. B. (1992). *Organizational architecture*. San Francisco: Jossey-Bass.

Nelson, E. C., Batalden, P. B., Huber, T. P., Godfrey, M. M., Headrick. L. A., & Wasson, J. H. (2002, September). Microsystems in healthcare: Part I. Learning from high-performing front-line clinical units. *Joint Commission Journal on Quality Improvement. 28*(9). 472–493.

Newell, L. M., & Christensen, D. (n.d.). Who's counting now? ROI for patient safety IT intiatives. Retrieved February 1, 2011, from http://www.auburn.edu/~burnsma/HADM4970/classroom/JHIM/17-4/newell.pdf

National Quality Forum. (2010). *Safe practices for better healthcare—2010 update: A consensus report*. Retrieved May 28, 2010 from http://www.qualityforum.org/Publications/2009/03/Safe_Practices_for_Better_Healthcare–2009_Update.aspx

Robert Wood Johnson Foundation. (2001). *With hospitals, it's survival of the fattest: Not the fittest*. Retrieved May 22, 2010, from http://www.rwjf.org/reports/grr/028054.htm

Schein, E. H. (1984, January 15). Leadership and organizational Studies; Coming to a new awareness of organizational culture. *MIT Sloan Management Review*. Retrieved January 30, 2011, from http://sloan review.mit.edu/the-magazine/articles/1984/winter/2521/coming-to-a-new-awareness-of-organizational-culture/?purchase=yes/

Senge, P. M. (1990). *The fifth discipline: The art & practice of the learning organization*. New York: Doubleday.

Senge, P. M. (2004). *Peter Senge comments on "Illuminating the blind spot: leadership in the context of emerging worlds"* Retrieved January 30, 2011, from http://www.enhyper.com/content/leadership.pdf

Shaw, C. D. (2003). Editorial: Evaluating accreditation. *International Journal for Quality in Health Care, 15*(6), pp. 455–456.

Trivedi, V. (n.d.). *Learning organizations: An overview*. Retrieved May 25, 2010, from http://www.indianmba.com/Faculty_Column/FC1092/fc1092.html

Weatherly, L. A. (2003). Human capital the elusive asset: Measuring and managing human capital: A strategic imperative for HR. *HR Magazine*. Retrieved May 22, 2010, from BNET database http://findarticles.com/p/articles/mi_m3495/is_3_48/ai_98830435/pg_7/?tag=content;col

Wheatley, M. J. (1999). *Leadership and the new science: Discovering order in a chaotic world*. San Francisco, CA: Berret-Koehler.

9

Design at the Leadership Level (System Level)

OVERVIEW

Nelson et al. (2002) emphasized leadership as one of the key elements necessary to achieve high levels of performance in microsystems. They emphasized leadership as the anchor to maintain constancy of purpose, establish clear goals, and promote a positive culture.

According to Botnick, Bisognano, and Haraden (2006), leadership is the essential element to implement patient safety, and these tasks cannot be delegated. Leaders have authority and span of control, and they greatly influence the organizational culture. Leaders hold the compass that guides staff on which direction to follow. It is a moral compass, a strategic compass, and a values compass. The leader is able to guide staff in a completely different direction than they are used to, or in which they feel comfortable. Leaders have the capacity to "change the way we do things around here."

Leaders must keep the staff's attention on a shared vision, create a sense of meaning about their work, build trust through consistent behaviors, and possess a strong belief and awareness in their abilities—which also creates in others a tendency to follow and do likewise (Bennis & Nanus, 1985). It is up to the leadership to set the course through role modeling a value system, developing and implementing strategic plans, and aligning the organizational steps and resources for the development, implementation, and sustainability of patient safety practices that reduce and/or eliminate risk of harm to patients and to staff.

The governing board is accountable for the quality and patient safety of the health care organization. As such, they need to be strong patient advocates and see the health care system through the eyes of the patients and their families. It is common knowledge that health care workers make the worst patients. Why? Because they know all of the potential things that can go wrong and do go wrong on a daily basis. From the minute patients are admitted to the hospital, their risk for harm increases, and the Medicare population is even more at risk.

HealthGrades is the leading independent health care ratings company that provides health care ratings for hospitals, nursing homes, and physicians. In 2010, HealthGrades reported its *Seventh Annual Patient Safety Study in American Hospitals*. There were 958,202 total patient safety events affecting 39.5 million Medicare admissions. The report estimated that 96,413 deaths could be directly attributed to a patient safety event. This translates into Medicare patients having a 1-in-10 chance of dying when a medical error is experienced. Also, there were large safety gaps between the top performing versus lower performing hospitals. Medicare patients who were treated at hospitals with a HealthGrades Patient Safety Excellence Award had on average 43 percent lower risk of experiencing 1 or more of the 15 patient safety events studied, compared to patients treated at bottom-ranked hospitals.

For board members to become passionate about patient safety, they have to recognize their own accountabilities and also know what their role is in making health care safer. More than ever do governing boards use storytelling of patients' experiences as part of their quality and patient safety briefings. This method assists board members to see patients not just as numbers on a dashboard but as people whose lives are profoundly affected by the care provided to them.

PATIENT SAFETY WALKROUNDS

In the 1980s, after Peters and Waterman published *In Search of Excellence*, management by walking around became popular. In effect, leadership became visible. Leaders interacted with and listened to frontline staff through informal encounters, which allowed them to see how processes were done on a daily basis and provide support where and when it was needed.

Frankel et al. (2003) extended the concept and created Patient Safety Leadership WalkRounds, which involve the senior leadership conducting regular weekly rounds to the various areas of the hospital. The senior team engages staff at the unit level to discuss adverse events or near misses as well as the system factors that led to them. They ask questions such as, "Were you able to care for your patients as safely as possible? If not, why not?" A database is developed from this information, categorizing the various issues reported along with prioritizing the actions taken by the leadership, and results are shared throughout the organization.

WalkRounds are also attached to the peer review process as much for peer review protection as part of quality improvement efforts. Staff realize that they feel safe by reporting events to the leadership. These rounds serve as a catalyst for changing the patient safety climate at the unit level as well as stimulating learning at both the board and the unit level.

Many continuous improvement projects are identified and acted on with frontline staff and leadership assigned to handle them, with target dates for accomplishing their aims.

These rounds provide the leadership with a "fresh eye" for seeing how their budgetary decisions impact the work done on a daily basis by staff working on the front line. These rounds also provide the staff working at the unit level with a chance to have a voice when sharing concerns about patient safety without fear of reprisal or punishment. Over time, trust develops as the values of the leadership are translated into actions that, like the leadership, become visible.

Patient Safety Leadership WalkRounds may be supportive for one of the organizational factors associated with high performance in quality and safety in academic medical centers. Keroack et al. (2007) emphasized that shared sense of purpose, a hands-on leadership style, and accountability systems with focus on results combined with a culture of collaboration are key qualities shared by top performers on measures of safety, mortality, clinical effectiveness, and equity of care for 79 academic medical centers. Also, these leadership behaviors and organizational practices were associated with measurable differences in patient-level measures of quality and safety.

LEADERSHIP VISION

According to Senge (1990), when people truly share a vision, they are committed to it, and that commitment creates a connectedness to others with shared aspirations. A vision becomes a powerful motivator to create future realities.

One compelling example of a shared vision occurs in the film "Apollo 13," where the leader of the team has a compelling vision: get the astronauts home safely. "Failure is not an option," he states: a quote attributed to Gene Kranz, lead flight director then for Mission Control (Keppler Speakers, n.d.).

Peter Senge emphasizes on shared vision because, if people don't have a compelling desire to achieve the same thing, the forces in support of maintaining the status quo can be overwhelming. Shared visions also foster innovation through risk-taking and experimentation. When new things are tried for achieving one's goal—some work, some don't, and it is a learning process.

Visions are compelling and keep the momentum forward moving. Staff is motivated to take risks to achieve the shared vision. The leadership determines the boundaries for risk-taking. One shared vision for patient safety is to reduce or eliminate harm to patients. There should be a safe environment for everyone that includes reducing or eliminating harm to staff as well.

According to IHI, the vision of health care in the future involves these six aims: safe, effective, timely, efficient, equitable, and patient centered combined with the "no needless" list of:

No needless deaths

No needless pain or suffering

No helplessness in those served or serving

No unwanted waiting

No waste

No one left out (Institute for Healthcare Improvement [IHI], n.d.).

Leaders in health care must strive for zero preventable deaths and zero adverse events for patients and for staff.

CULTURE

Does organizational culture impact patient safety management? Chiu, Pan, and Wei (2008) examined the relationship between organizational culture and patient safety management. Chiu et al. studied four categories of organizational culture (rational, developmental, group, and hierarchical). Rational culture emphasizes the external environmental issues rather than internal issues. The organization's focus is on economic considerations, competitiveness, and productivity. Developmental culture stresses flexibility and external focus is on individualism, risk taking, and innovation. Group culture stresses management through teamwork and staff development. The environment is humanistic and empowering.

Hierarchical stresses adherence to following rules and regulations as well as authority and responsibilty. There is emphasis on operational controls. They concluded that group culture had a strong influence on safety management, whereas rational culture had a negative impact on safety management. Group culture was cited as the most significant predictor of safety management. They recommended building a group culture by implementing participatory management, delegating authority, team building, strengthening worker participation, developing human resources methods, and using open communication styles.

PURPOSE

Why do we get out of bed in the morning? A sense of purpose is a powerful motivator. There is a certain spirituality in purpose that transcends the mundane tasks and provides a real sense of accomplishment and satisfaction when a job is well done.

Leider (2004) describes purpose as "the quality we want to center our work around: the way we orient ourselves toward life and work. It is the way we make sense or meaning about our lives. . . . Purpose is the recognition of the presence of the sacred within us and the choice of work that is consistent with that presence."

Having a sense of purpose enhances worker engagement and connectedness to others and to the organization as a whole.

Commins (2010) reported the results of a survey of more than 235,000 employees from nearly 400 hospitals. He reported that older employees—those born in 1945 or earlier—tend to be the most satisfied group, whereas younger employees are the least satisfied group. Both groups need to receive recognition and be included in decisions. Commins also reported that 45 percent of hospital employees feel distanced from or discontent in their current work.

The survey indicated a strong correlation between patient satisfaction and employee partnership. This means that there is an essential need for hospital leadership to ensure that employees feel empowered and engaged for patients to be satisfied with their care. Employee dissatisfaction can lead to a disengaged workforce in which patient safety efforts are difficult to implement. Also, a unit with a high turnover rate may be at a higher risk for adverse events to occur because new employees experience a learning curve as they acclimate to the numerous policies, procedures, and expected communication among the various departments, groups, and staff.

Vahey, Aiken, Sloane, Sean, and Vargas (2004) reported that more than 40 percent of hospital staff nurses score in the high range for job-related burnout, and more than 1 in 5 hospital staff nurses stated that they intend to leave their current hospital jobs within 1 year. Burnout was measured by feelings of emotional exhaustion and lack of personal accomplishment. This study also supported previous studies with positive correlation between nursing satisfaction and patient satisfaction. Vahey et al. reported that patients who were cared for on units where nurses perceived that they had adequate staffing, good administrative support for nursing care, and good relationships with physicians and other nurses were more than twice as likely as other patients to report high satisfaction with their care. Also, nurses reported significantly lower burnout on these units.

This study also provided linkage between nursing burnout levels and patient satisfaction scores. After adjustment was made for patient characteristics, patients who were cared for by nurses who experienced higher than average levels of emotional exhaustion were only half as likely to be highly satisfied with their nursing care as patients who were cared for by nurses with lower than average emotional exhaustion.

In health care, it is odd that although the mission of many hospitals is to provide quality care to patients and families, those hospitals do not always weave that same philosophy into their staff culture. One nurse shared with me a story about mandatory overtime:

> Mandatory overtime made me feel like I was just a number to fill in for someone who called in sick. You never knew when this was going to happen. At best, I knew it was my turn for mandatory overtime next; at worst, it came as a surprise. There was no regard for my life, my personal commitments to my family. I felt treated like a number to fill in the space on the scheduling sheet.

Leadership must convey a sense of purpose to staff on a consistent basis. Silos and favored departments and groups must yield to building cross-functional teams at the unit level whose purpose is clear. The IOM in *Crossing the Quality Chasm: A New Health System for the 21st Century* (2001) outlined six aims for improvement of the health care system.

- *Safe*: Health care needs to avoid injuries to patients and to staff.
- *Effective*: Results need to be based on current scientific knowledge and should refrain from overuse and underuse of services.
- *Timely*: The right care needs to be provided at the right time, reducing delays and waits.

- *Efficient*: Waste needs to be avoided in equipment, supplies, ideas, and energy.
- *Equitable*: Uniform care must be provided with no variation in quality due to gender, ethnic group, geographic location, and/or socio-economic status.
- *Patient centered*: Care needs to be provided in a manner that is respectful and also responsive to individual patient preferences, needs, and values. The values of the patient need to guide all clinical decision making.

Leadership at the unit level who work in cross-functional teams need to have a clear sense of purpose that each patient under their team's care on that day will receive care that is safe, effective, timely, efficient, equitable, and patient centered.

Leaders, both formal and informal, exist at all levels within an organization. Frontline leaders who are empowered to make decisions that are in alignment with the organization's mission and vision can be very powerful and effective catalysts for providing quickly adaptable, responsive actions that are needed for both quality and patient safety in today's complex health care systems.

LEADERSHIP STYLE

Is there a leadership style that has a positive effect on patient safety culture, initiatives, and outcomes? McFadden, Hengan, and Gowen (2009) used structural equation modeling obtained from a national survey of over 200 hospitals to investigate the existence of a patient safety chain in hospitals. The authors utilized high reliability organization theory, multifactor leadership theory, and literature on total quality management concepts. The elements included in their patient safety chain consisted of transformational leadership, patient safety culture, patient safety initiatives, and patient safety outcomes. They hypothesized that transformational leadership is based on a combination of charisma and inspiration. This study provided empirical evidence of a patient safety chain. Improving patient safety begins at the top of the patient chain with the CEO's who possess a transformational leadership style which is directly related to patient safety culture. The patient safety culture is tied to successful implementation of patient safety initiatives and finally, to patient safety outcomes. Certainly, more research in this area is called for.

ROLE MODELING AND MENTORING

Leaders are expected, to paraphrase Mahatma Gandhi, "to be the change they wish to see." For good or for bad, they lead by example. Eventually, the leader's behavior traits influence the behaviors of all levels and categories of staff. Ambler (2007) calls this the "viral" impact of leadership. To implement and sustain a patient safety culture, the influence of leadership cannot be underestimated.

Every organization has a collective consciousness. Some staff tend to demonstrate patterns of behavior that rise or sink "only to the level of the water they are swimming in." The leadership determines the water level.

A role model has observable behaviors to which others would like to aspire. Role models influence the values, attitudes, and behaviors of others in the organization.

What kinds of behaviors should we expect to see to transform health care from its present state into one that is safe, effective, timely, efficient, equitable, and patient centered?

Think about leaders and other staff who have inspired us to become better persons—leaders who inspired us to be part of work projects in which we felt a real sense of accomplishment and pride; leaders who listened and supported us with empathy and genuine concern; or leaders who expressed their vision with real passion that was infectious. People possess different levels of maturity, caring, communication skills, analytical skills, and emotional skills.

The ability to create and sustain meaningful relationships where dialogue is exchanged, genuine caring is expressed, differences are expected and expressed with respect for person, combined with competence and clear sense of direction, are all characteristics for further study to see how they may enhance a patient safety culture.

What characteristics in leaders are predictive of success?

Kaplan (2008) addressed the University of Chicago School of Business at its convocation ceremony, by reporting on research pertaining to 300 detailed assessments and rating of the candidates on more than 30 specific abilities in firms funded by private equity investors.

The ratings on the specific abilities were compared to subsequent success. Success was measured from evaluations on actual performance and the investment's financial return.

Kaplan reported that the most successful Chief Executive Officers (CEOs) were persistent, efficient, and proactive (PEP). For buyouts, Kaplan reported that CEOs who scored high on PEP succeeded

75 to 90 percent of the time compared to CEOs who did not score high on PEP, who succeeded less than 50 percent of the time. Kaplan concluded his speech with these words:

> The piece of advice that goes with this is to choose work you like to do with people you respect. It is difficult to be persistent, efficient, and proactive when you don't like what you are doing and don't respect the people you are working with.

There is a paucity of research in the area of role modeling and effects on aspects of patient safety.

One area in which some research has been conducted is in the area of hand hygiene. Pittet (2001) stated that hospital-acquired infections affect approximately 5 to 10 percent of all hospitalized patients and are the most common cause of preventable morbidity and mortalities. Even though hand hygiene prevents cross-infection in hospitals, health care workers' adherence to guidelines remains poor. Compliance with hand hygiene is usually estimated as below 50 percent (Pittet, 2001).

Pittet et al. (2004) reported results of a cross-sectional study that directly observed and surveyed 163 physicians at a large university hospital about current practices and beliefs. They reported that only approximately 57 percent of physicians adhered to hand hygiene, with wide variation across medical specialties. They reported that adherence to hand hygiene was associated with the belief of being a role model for other colleagues. Also associated with adherence to hand hygiene practices was availability of hand-rub solution and a positive attitude toward the practice of hand hygiene after patient contact.

Recently, Schnieder et al. (2009) reported results from a prospective observational study within pediatric and cardiac intensive care of a tertiary care children's hospital. They observed and recorded the following hand hygiene adherence for two critical care fellows and four nurse orienteers. They reported that the adherence of junior practitioners improved under the supervision of adherent role models, with an average increase of 34 percentage points, from 22 percent of 200 hand hygiene opportunities to 56 percent of 234 hand hygiene opportunities, as a result of role modeling. These results strongly suggested that hand hygiene behavior role modeled by senior practitioners critically influenced the behaviors of other staff.

Dracup and Bryan-Brown (2004) wrote in an editorial that the concept of mentoring, although established in the business world, was still new to nursing. They cited the five core competencies developed for the RWJF Executive Nurse Fellows Program for leaders and mentors to be used for establishing mentor programs. The five competencies were:

- *Self-knowledge*: This includes not only knowing one's strengths and weaknesses in the context of the demands and challenges of the organization but also knowing one's own learning style.
- *Strategic vision*: Strategic vision is the ability to connect the dots from scanning the environment and identify critical trends in the external environment for decision making.
- *Risk-taking and creativity*: This refers to the ability to turn lemons into lemonade. It requires going outside the traditional solutions and providing novel and innovative solutions. It includes the ability to turn mistakes into opportunities for learning and growth.
- *Interpersonal and communication effectiveness*: This is related to balance. The partnership is equal and not power- and control-related. The relationship is one of respect, honest communication, and engagement.
- *Inspiration*: Mentors provide a positive framework. Mentors are change agents who create personal and organizational change in a manner that addresses resistance; they build teams that move resistance to positive actions.

Role modeling and mentoring are interrelated. The person who is being mentored looks at the mentor as a role model. The leaders shape the environment in which patient safety resides. New physicians and nurses bring with them into the system their past experiences (either for the good or bad), and they play out behaviors learned daily in the workplace.

KNOWLEDGE

The leaders influence the patient safety culture. To develop and sustain a patient safety culture, the leaders need to be competent in concepts related to human factors, communication, teamwork, use of evidence-based practice, reporting systems, just culture, and application of quality improvement concepts. Leaders in health care must have the right knowledge, skills, and attitude to handle the complexities of health care in the 21st century. Without having core competencies related to patient safety, the leaders cannot implement and sustain a patient safety culture.

REWARD AND RECOGNITION

Reward and recognition are used in health care organizations to motivate staff when implementing business goals and objectives. When patient safety initiatives are being implemented, the leadership has to decide what actions will provide the desired outcomes for patient safety.

Monetary rewards can be a motivator for higher productivity in the workplace, but only to a point; if the money is not enough, it can be a dissatisfier. However, a greater motivator for workers is experiencing personal fulfillment and realizing that their work has purpose and that it is recognized by the organization.

In the 2009 book, *Drive: The Surprising Truth About What Motivates Us*, author Daniel Pink asserts that people have an innate inner drive to be autonomous, self-determined, and connected to one another. Pink presents Google's Results-Only Work Environment (ROWE), where employees get to work on whatever project they choose for 20 percent of the time. Google is cited by Pink as an example of ROWE, in which innovations are developed, such as Gmail.

Even more radical is the notion that each employee is autonomous and works on what he or she wants, from wherever he or she wants, with meetings as optional, as long as the work aims for the results are defined by the company.

Rewards used for cognitive challenges tend to narrow the focus and stifle creativity. Some flaws in assigning monetary rewards include decreasing productivity, stifling creativity, stimulating cheating and taking shortcuts to win, and instigating shortsighted thinking. Rewards for simple tasks that have a clear goal may be effective; however, when there are cognitive challenges involved, higher incentives lead to poorer performance. Pink posits that businesses don't need to do more of the wrong thing; the carrot and stick mechanistic approach to rewards will not be very effective for today's challenges. Traditional notions of management will gain compliance but not engagement.

Unless the leadership provides vision and purpose that is reinforced with appropriate rewards and recognition that stimulate employees to be engaged and motivated, it fails.

Intrinsic rewards are the rewards that inspire excitement, and keep an employee working beyond what is usually expected to overcome challenges in pursuing something worthwhile.

Implementation of patient safety initiatives requires teamwork on a daily basis; therefore, when rewards are being constructed, the power of using intrinsic versus extrinsic motivators should be considered.

Extrinsic motivators are external: someone else is trying to make you do something; intrinsic is when you want to do something yourself.

According to a Gallup Poll, the number one motivator was public praise and recognition (D'Ausillo, 2008). The Gallup Poll also stated that when workers are actively disengaged, they miss more days of work and are less loyal to employers. This can be very costly.

Deeprose (2007) reported that team reward systems have now become the norm for organizations that have self-managed or at least semi-autonomous work teams. In many companies, team rewards are directly linked with productivity increases of the team or organization. The author stated that many of these team-based companies have also developed ways to measure and reward teams for their progress in sharing information, working together, communicating across teams, and skill development. The critical component of this is measurement that ensures valid and reliable benchmarks to gauge progress.

Recognition can be simple things such as bringing enthusiasm, recognizing publicly the team's accomplishments, taking pictures of great teamwork and posting them in public places, writing thank-you letters, and marking milestones with mini-celebrations. Individual rewards should be centered on the individual's contribution to the team's goals. Examples include assisting a team member, filling in for a team member who is sick, coming up with a novel solution to a team problem, teaching a new skill to others, or volunteering to perform a time-consuming task.

LEADERSHIP ATTRIBUTES

According to Kreitner (2007), leadership "is the process of inspiring, influencing, and guiding others to participate in a common effort."

Executive leaders in health care make decisions that have the potential to impact the entire system's performance. Design of the leadership is an essential element in the Myers Model for Patient Safety and Accreditation because, as Bennis (1985) states:

> Leaders are people who do the right thing; managers are people who do things right.

The values and ethics of leadership guide the behaviors and the decision-making process on a daily basis. Leaders influence the culture of the entire organization, which includes the patient safety culture.

Leaders in health care organizations face new challenges that frequently test their character. According to Bennis (1999), character is essential to leadership. Bennis stated that research conducted at Harvard University indicated that 85 percent of the leader's performance depended on his or her personal character. Character was described as the inner voice that acknowledges the real self as a fully integrated human being. Character in executive leaders includes drive, competence, and integrity. Unfortunately, there are many executives who lack the moral compass that guides them to place their organizational goals ahead of their personal goals.

The Center for Creative Leadership's survey included 2,200 leaders working in 15 organizations from 2006 to 2008 and was reported in 2009. This research identified the following seven core competencies as most critical to the leader's current and future success:

- How well the leader directs and motivates staff
- How well the leader translates vision into feasible and attainable business strategies
- How well the leader transitions the organization through change
- How well the leader recognizes and rewards staff achievements
- How well the leader works effectively with others in top management
- How well the leader perseveres under adverse conditions
- How quickly the leader learns new technical or business knowledge

What happens when the person selected for a leadership role does not have "the right stuff"? Anderson (2008) reported that the American Management Association (AMA) estimated that it costs 3.5 times the annual salary of a departed employee to replace him or her. This study was not at the executive level. What if a key member of the executive team (and they are all key members) makes bad decisions that have been costly or create an environment that does not promote collaboration and cooperation? These impacts may be hidden for a while and are difficult to quantify; however, they have the potential to be very costly, and the full effects may take years to play out in the organization.

VALUES, ETHICS, AND DECISION MAKING

Without the right values and ethics, followers cannot respect or trust that their leaders will do the right thing every time. Values and ethics are embedded in leaders who role model correct behaviors on a daily basis. Behaving ethically means that the behaviors are consistent with what is right or moral. Values and ethics are the core of any health care organization. Core values of a health care system are usually stated in terms such as integrity, teamwork, caring, and professionalism. Values guide expected behaviors. Values are also what the organization judges to be right. As such, values become the moral compass for ethical decision making.

Example: The hospital's administrator leaves early every day because he wants to avoid the traffic jam. He takes a hands-off approach to quality and patient safety. When the patient safety manager tries to get the hospital administrator to participate in patient safety rounds, his reply is, "I support you 100 percent in patient safety; you can represent me in my absence."

Although the hospital has stated that it has taken a nonpunitive approach to patient safety, the hospital administrator has reversed two decisions made by the patient safety team and has issued written warnings for honest mistakes when the patient experienced harm.

The staff has stated to the patient safety manager that they are afraid to report because they do not trust that the hospital administrator will adhere to the patient safety policy.

EXAMPLE: FLY WITH ME

In April 2010, Southwest Airlines ranked #4 among airlines and #12 among all industries listed in *Fortune* magazine's annual list of the world's Most Admired Companies (Southwest, n.d.).

Gittel (2003) studied Southwest a Airlines for its ability to build and sustain high performance relationships among managers, employees, unions, and suppliers. Southwest employees were observed to have high levels of shared goals, shared knowledge, and mutual respect. There was recognition among the employees that every job had equal importance. No one department was more special or more important than another department. Employees are encouraged to openly recognize major events in the lives of employees and families.

Leadership follows the principle of being credible, consistent, and caring. There is emphasis on frontline leadership, and Southwest has more supervisors per frontline employee than any other airline.

Southwest's principles applied to the leadership in a health care organization may be effective in developing a higher satisfied workforce and may assist in developing and sustaining a patient safety culture.

LEADERSHIP DECISION MAKING

Decision making occurs at all levels in the organization, from the board room to the frontline staff. The quality of the decisions depends on the decision-making process, in which there is wide variation. The variation in the quality of decision making affects patient safety. Decisions that are made today may take years to take full effect in the system. Of course, everyone brings their own values and views to the decision-making process.

Senge (1990) spoke about mental models as key to building a learning organization. Sometimes decisions are based exclusively on the leader's unique view of the world and his or her authority to decide upon a course of actions—and this can occur without the leader fully listening to others. Two people can see the same event and come away with entirely different perceptions of, and assumptions about, the event.

Assumptions are not truth and many times our assumptions are incorrect. When one assumes that only his or her view is correct, then the only task wanting is clear: get others on board. This excludes dialogue and learning. The decision has already been made. Meaningful dialogue generates from mutual trust and respect rather than from power. Authority to make a decision, however, does not guarantee that it is the right decision.

Combining skills in advocacy and inquiry increases the likelihood that others will commit to action. Advocacy is about making views known to others. This is done by supporting your view with rational statements. Other people are encouraged to explore any gaps they may perceive in your view.

Inquiry is about how questions are posed. It allows people to probe into one another's reasoning to understand the conclusions they have reached.

Garvin and Roberto (2001) stated that there is considerable evidence showing that when groups consider many alternatives they engage in more thoughtful discussions and usually avoid making hasty decisions by settling on an easy or obvious answer. Assumption testing is part of this process. They emphasized that poor listening skills produces flawed analysis and also personal friction. Sometimes, there is a blatant unwillingness to acknowledge the facts and opinions of others. To develop an effective patient safety culture requires thoughtful dialogue and excellent communication skills. Leaders should assess their own communication skills to enable them to actively keep staff engaged in patient safety initiatives.

Day and Schoemaker (2004) added that the periphery should be ignored at our peril. Monitoring of the periphery can help to diffuse small problems before they escalate into larger problems or crisis. Problems in the workplace appear first at the borders, at the front line.

In some organizations, when the middle manager or frontline staff tries to convey bad news to the leaders, he or she can be labeled as the problem and in the worst-case scenario, may have to leave the organization. Others quickly observe the behaviors and keep quiet rather than suffer the same consequences.

This is analogous to a day at the beach. People are sitting on the beach, hidden beneath the umbrellas. There is a lifeguard on a high tower that sets boundaries for the swimmers in the water. When one of the swimmers ventures too far into the deep waters, the sound of a shrill whistle echoes in the air. The people sitting safely under their umbrellas on the beach can hear the shrill whistle. When new people enter the beach, they are warned, "Don't go out into the deep water; the lifeguard is watching."

The same holds true for health care organizations. As new employees enter the system, the existing staff warn them about what behaviors are acceptable and what behaviors will get them into trouble. The leadership sets the behavior boundaries.

If staff is afraid to speak up because of the "kill the messenger" syndrome, the leadership becomes very vulnerable, as does the organization, which is collectively in denial.

It is well known that transparency is necessary for the health care organization to learn. If staff does not report adverse events, these opportunities to reduce risk are lost.

DECISIONS ON ORGANIZATIONAL STRUCTURES

There is no "one size fits all" in terms of best fit for organizational structures. Each has its advantages and disadvantages.

Divisional structures divide the organization's operations into product/service or customer segments or even geographic locations (Borkowski, 2009). Divisional structures in hospitals have created silos of competitive departments and groups, frequently not in tune with overall organizational goals. Communication occurs more in a top-down sequence than in a lateral sequence that permeates across the various departments, groups, and/or locations. Two types of organizational structures that may assist with breaking down silos and increasing adaptation ability are the matrix and organic structures.

Matrix organizational structures assign priority to functional activities and product lines at the same time (Smith & Flarey, 1999). Both product and functional structures are implemented at the same time in each department. One example would be creating a vertical functional structure for patient care services, ancillary and plant services, human resources, finance, medical staff, and managed care, and then establishing horizontal, team-based structures that cross the traditional functional reporting boundaries.

Each organization would create its own matrix based on individual needs; however, the team structures would assist with breaking down silos and would facilitate integration for a full continuum of services. Matrix organizations have dual-reporting relationships instead of the more traditional linear management structure. There is also an implied matrix structure when staff is assigned to be on interdisciplinary work teams. They report to the team leader and to their functional managers. Matrix organizations have been criticized for having potential role confusion.

Organic structures are structures that are decentralized and loosely defined. There is a lot of lateral communication and much greater individual autonomy. Organic structures are purpose driven, and staff is empowered to do their work. There is a connected workforce that has diversity and capacity for agility, growth, and innovation (Burns & Stalker, n.d.).

Hospitals with organic structures allow greater innovation and responsiveness when caring for patients, one patient at a time. Large sample sizes and control studies are not mandatory to assess if care can be improved at the bedside, one patient at a time.

Self-directed work units that comprise cross disciplines should form, inform, and disband as needed to provide holistic care to patients, improve processes, and continually learn from mistakes made.

In organic structures, the leadership at the center is anchored by values, purpose, and collective intelligence. Leaders at the unit level are mentors and guides and follow the pattern of values and purpose expressed by the core leadership. For patient safety, the organic structures would enable agility, adaptability, and responsiveness at the front line where patient care is provided. There would be greater autonomy for decision making at the front line. Staff follow the six aims for the health care system for decision making: safe, effective, timely, efficient, equitable, and patient centered.

DECISIONS ON ENVIRONMENTAL DESIGN

How do health care leaders structure the environment to enhance the use of teams, build a patient safety culture, and decrease or eliminate adverse events?

Environments need to be enhanced in a manner that optimizes use of technology and design to reduce risk to patients and promotes interdisciplinary teamwork. To reduce the number of adverse events, standardized and adaptable patient room environments may be created in which each patient has his or her own room large enough to accommodate family members to assist with care. The rooms might be designed in a manner that allows acuity adaptability when needed so that the right skill level comes to the patient at the right time.

There should be a decentralized approach for patient care. This might mean envisioning interdisciplinary office areas, break rooms, and lounge rooms for staff and creating spaces that allow for higher interaction among the various disciplines with patients and their families and/or significant others.

Some future examples include use of robotics for patient care rounding, use of radio-frequency identification tags that track every health care provider and piece of equipment to allow quicker responses in emergencies, and to enhance patient flow efforts.

Smart beds that transmit patients' physiological vital signs to the team and alert the team when individualized patient thresholds have been exceeded may be available. There will be increased use of technology for remote monitoring in patients' homes as well, and telemedicine will continue to expand (Andrews, 2009).

Patients are a key part of any health care process. Patients should be allowed to document questions for the health care team to answer in the patients' medical record. There would also be an area for the team's response to them.

DECISIONS ON MODELS OF CARE

Among the increasing numbers of patient-centered models of care is the one called Planetree. The Planetree model is a patient-centered model that brings patients and families into active participation in their plan of care. The environment integrates nature into a healing environment (Planetree, n.d.).

The Planetree model is an excellent example of a vision turned into purpose, then strategy, followed by implementation of structures and processes that support the vision, strategy, and purpose. Since implementing Planetree in 1992, Griffin Hospital, in Derby, Connecticut, receives consistently high patient satisfaction scores. Griffin Hospital was also honored with a 10th year on *Fortune's Best Companies to Work For* list in 2009 (Griffin Hospital, 2009).

A nursing practice environment model of care that is recognized nationally is the Magnet model. The Magnet Recognition program was developed by the American Nurses Credentialing Center (ANCC) to recognize organizations that possess nursing excellence. Hospitals that have achieved Magnet Status receive higher scores in the *U.S. News & World Report* for America's best hospitals (ANCC, n.d.). Magnet hospitals attract nurses who choose to join them because of the enriched work environment. The work environment is one in which nurses are recognized and rewarded. Professional nursing practice is embodied within an enriched practice environment. There are 14 attributes that make these organizations stand out as the embodiment of professionalism and excellence in nursing practice. These attributes (called forces) shape the system's conceptual framework for nursing practice.

Magnet recognition status for nursing staff may become an expectation by consumers. Nurses who work in Magnet hospitals have higher satisfaction levels and less turnovers, plus patients have decreased mortality and increased satisfaction levels (Lundmark, n.d.).

Laschinger and Heather (2006) tested a theoretical model linking conditions within a professional nursing practice environment with patient safety outcomes. They concluded that patient safety outcomes are related to the quality of the work environment for nurses, with staffing adequacy directly affecting nurses' emotional exhaustion. One of the primary roles of nursing leadership is to ensure that the nursing practice environment decreases nurse burnout, which in turn decreases adverse events.

DECISIONS ON NURSING MODELS OF CARE

Innovative nursing models will be needed to provide care in the future. The design of these models will enable patients to better self-manage their disease by becoming active participants in their daily care. This should translate into less utilization of emergency rooms and need of acute stays with the potential to reduce adverse events. RWJF's white paper (2008) reported on 24 innovative nursing models. They stated that over half of the 24 innovative nursing models studies deployed an interdisciplinary team for care delivery and for inpatients; this translated into nursing leading teams of interdisciplinary providers as well as ancillary staff.

It was also reported that 6 of the 24 innovative care delivery models included using the home as an alternative setting of care for individuals who normally would be admitted to a hospital or a long-term care unit.

The common theme in almost half of the 24 models was the active engagement of the patient and his or her family that enhanced patient self-management of his or her disease process. Use of new technology was reported in over half of the new models as well. Another example cited was the use of telepharmacy-dispensing machines for prescription medications in remote Alaskan villages supplemented by consultations with pharmacists directly using Internet-based technology. Many of the innovative models stated their goals to be patient satisfaction, lower costs, and improved patient and fiscal outcomes.

LEADERSHIP DECISIONS FOR SELF-MANAGED TEAMS

Self-managed teams may integrate the leadership and management functions in the future at the unit level. How self-managed teams perform and communicate with each other influences the culture of patient safety and may reduce adverse events.

According to Rivera (2010), autonomous work-group designs are best suited to situations in which there are no major barriers to sharing knowledge among all of the group members. Also, the tasks to be accomplished are routine. Work environments in which tasks are unstable and require the application of highly specialized skill sets or knowledge are not conducive to group members acquiring skills and learning from each other. The team members need to have a common understanding of the team's work processes.

Successful self-managed teams do not just happen. Rami, C. (2010). agreeed with the previous work of Zawacki and Norman (1994) and discussed five stages of self-managed teams' evolution.

It starts with the typical hospital structure (hierarchical) and the leader provides one-on-one supervision.

The leader evolves into the group manager, who now transitions to the team coordinator, mentor, and coach.

The group manager becomes the team coordinator and provides a structure for the self-managed team members to receive the training they need to assume more of the leadership tasks.

The team assumes many of the duties previously done by the group manager.

The group manager (e.g., team coordinator) now becomes the key resource for the team.

Two training programs that enhance team performance are the Team STEPPS, mentioned briefly in the previous chapter, and Comprehensive Unit-Based Safety Program (CUSP). Team STEPPS was developed by the U.S. Department of Defense with collaboration of Agency for Healthcare Research and Quality (AHRQ) in 2006. The program's goal was to improve communication and teamwork skills among the various groups of health care professionals by use of evidence-based curriculum for training.

AHRQ (2006) reported that Abington Memorial Hospital implemented the Team STEPPS with other initiatives. Results included a 27 percent decline in patient adverse events as measured by the Global Trigger Tool and a 30 percent decrease in crude mortality rate.

According to AHRQ (2008), a CUSP is "a safety culture program that is designed to educate and improve awareness about patient safety and quality of care, empower staff to take charge and improve safety in their workplace, create partnerships between units and hospital executives to improve organizational culture and provide resources for unit improvement efforts, and provide tools to investigate and learn from defects."

Staff come together for morning briefings, implement daily goals checklists, perform culture checkups, shadow other disciplines, and use ongoing measurement and feedback to improve teamwork and communication and improve the culture of safety.

For patient safety efforts there needs to be a focus on empowered teams working together to provide safe patient care at the unit level. This demands different organizational structures and cultures for transforming the workplace into one that possesses a patient safety culture.

Example: A registered nurse who works in an intensive care unit sees a physician not adhere to hand hygiene when he performs dressing changes. She states that the physician will just yell at her if she says anything. Nurses must be fully supported by administration and physician leaders to implement patient-centered care. Central line bundle checklists will not work if the nurses are afraid to speak up to the physician.

Staff are fearful to speak up when they see an action that becomes a risk point for the patient. Staff putting their egos as the priority instead of the needs of the patient should not be tolerated. Unfortunately, due to hierarchies, power gradients, and personalities, these types of unacceptable behaviors have been tolerated and accepted with silence.

Team training has proliferated, particularly for areas of high risk and fast pace such as operating rooms, emergency rooms, and labor and delivery areas. Team training assists staff with developing a better safety climate. All team training programs need to have measurements to evaluate the effectiveness of the training.

DECISIONS FOR TEAM TRAINING AT THE TOP

What about the leadership group? Sredl and Peng (2010) reported that nurse executive retention depended upon the nurse executive and the CEO to whom the nurse executive reports. The CEO's retention depends on maintaining good board relationships and a healthy economic performance. Nurse executives who do not maintain a healthy relationship with the CEO may be fired or forced to resign.

Nursing has a difficult time demonstrating healthy economic performance because nursing staff costs are an expense and not revenue producing. Nursing is the only department that provides 24/7 operations. Administration may tend to think of nursing only as the largest chunk of money for personnel costs, with approximately 75 percent of the hospital workforce directly under the nurse executive's authority.

Sredl and Peng cited studies that when the CEO leaves the organization, the nurse executive must forge a relationship with the new CEO, but he or she may not wish to do so. The new CEO might wish to bring his corporate base with him.

The authors also state that there is a paucity of research on the drivers and barriers to nursing job satisfaction affecting the turnover and retention decisions at the nurse executive level.

Turnover of nurse executives may prove to be an incalculable cost when the new nurse executive selected does not support the same values or agree with the strategic plans.

Because of the trend of nurse executives getting burned out and their average tenure decreasing, it is increasingly difficult to establish long-term relationships among members of the leadership group.

How well does the executive team function as a team? Do they actually work together within an equal partnership to achieve organizational goals? This area needs to be further explored in research. We know that the leadership shapes the culture and normative values for the health care organization. The complexity of health care with the scope of leadership roles creates an urgency to ensure that there is a team at the top that works effectively with each other and with the groups that are stakeholders in key processes within the organization.

Effective teamwork skills need to be role modeled from the top. The leadership walk-arounds at least make the executive group visible to staff. Also, leadership gets to see firsthand how their decisions affect the frontline staff on a daily basis.

Team training in the areas of communication, problem solving, conflict resolution, and negotiation skills are all essential leadership components. In the past, it was assumed that the leaders had these skills. When the leadership does not work well together, the dysfunctional behaviors tend to diffuse through the organization and play out with undesirable outcomes, which have implications for developing and/or sustaining a patient safety culture. Team training needs to be taken to a new level—the level at the top.

CONCLUSIONS

There needs to be the right leaders who role model the right behaviors and make the right decisions to ensure that patient care is safe, effective, timely, efficient, equitable, and patient centered. One leader's dysfunctional behaviors affect the entire organization. The complexity of health care requires that the leadership evaluate their current leadership design and decision making. Leaders must have the right values, ethics, and moral character to make the right decisions for patients and staff, especially when there are competing priorities.

There is no "one size fits all" for the type of organizational structures that will be successful for implementing patient safety programs; however, the development of teams at the microsystem level is essential to keep the workforce engaged. Group culture is supportive of a patient safety culture; leaner levels of management, use of multidisciplinary teams, and supportive human resource practices are recommended as building blocks to achieving a patient safety culture.

Nurse executives need to possess the right attributes that enable them to be successful members of a high performing team at the leadership level. Nurse executives shape the environment in which nurses provide care. Decisions need to be made regarding new nursing models of care. Also, there needs to be an assessment of the working environment in which nursing care is rendered. This assessment includes the formal and informal working structures, culture, and resources to ensure that nurses working on the front line have the leadership support necessary to provide safe and high quality care to patients.

REFERENCES

Agency for Healthcare Research and Quality. (2006). *Innovation profile: Team communication improvement initiatives enhance a hospital's culture of safety, leading to improved outcomes.* Retrieved May 30, 2010, from http://www.innovations.ahrq.gov/content.aspx?id=1783

Agency for Healthcare Research and Quality. (2008). *Unit-based safety program improves safety culture, reduces medication errors, and length of stay.* Retrieved May 30, 2010, from http://www.innovations.ahrq.gov/content.aspx?id=1769

Ambler, G. (2007). *The influence of leadership.* Retrieved June 1, 2010, from http://www.thepracticeofleadership.net/the-influence-of-leadership

American Nurses Credentialing Center. (n.d.). *Magnet overview.* Retrieved February 1, 2011, from http://www.nursecredentialing.org/Magnet/ProgramOverview.aspx

Anderson, D. (2008). *TKO Hiring: Ten knockout strategies for recruiting, interviewing, and hiring great people.* Hoboken, NJ: Wiley.

Andrews, M. (2009, July 15). *The high-tech hospital of the future: technology of all kinds is transforming the way medical systems work.* U.S. News & World Report. Retrieved May 20, 2010, from http://health.usnews.com/health-news/best-hospitals/articles/2009/07/15/the-high-tech-hospital-of-the-future.html

Bennis, W., & Nanus, B. (1985). *Leaders: Their strategies for taking charge.* New York: Harper & Row.

Bennis. W. (1999). The leadership advantage. Retrieved October 20, 2011 from http://www.hr-newcorp.com/articles/bennis_Leaders.pdf

Borkowski, N. (2009). *Organizational behavior, theory, and design in healthcare.* Sudbury, MA: Jones and Barlett Publishers.

Botnick, L, Bisognano, M., & Haraden, C. (2006). *Innovation series 2006: Leadership Guide to Patient Safety.* Retrieved May 28, 2010, from http://www.ihi.org/IHI/Topics/PatientSafety/SafetyGeneral/Literature/LeadershipGuidetoPatientSafety.htm

Burns, T., & Stalker, G. M. (n.d.). Mechanistic vs. organic organizational structure (contingency theory). Retrieved January 1, 2010, from http://www.businessmate.org/Article.php?ArtikelId=44

Center for Creative Leadership (CCL). (2009). *Research finds leadership skills inadequate to meet current and future demand.* The Practice of Leadership. Retrieved February 1, 2011 from http://www.thepracticeofleadership.net/2009/11/17/research-finds-leadership-skills-inadequate-to-meet-current-and-future-demand/

Chiu, C. H., Pan, W. H., & Wei, C. J. (2008). Does organizational culture impact patient safety management? *Asian Journal of Health and Information Sciences, 3*, 88–100.

Commins, J. (2010, June, 14). *Survey finds 45% of hospital employees discontented, disengaged.* Retrieved January 4, 2011 from http://www.healthleadersmedia .com/content/HR-252442/Survey-Finds-45-of-Hospital-Employees-Discontented-Disengaged

D'Ausillo, R. D. (2008). *What motivates your employees? Intrinsic vs. Extrinsic Rewards.* Retrieved May 24, 2010, from http://www.tmcnet.com/ channels/performance-management/articles/39417-what-motivates-employees-intrinsic-vs-extrinsic-rewards.htm

Day, G. S., & Schoemaker P. J. H. (2004). Driving through the fog: Managing at the edge. *Long Range Planning, 37*(4), 127–142.

Deeprose, D. (2007). *How to recognize and reward employees: 150 ways to inspire peak performance* (2nd ed.). New York: American Management Association.

Dracup, K., & Bryan-Brown, C. W. (2004). From novice to expert to mentor: Shaping the future. *American Journal of Critical Care, 13*, 448–450.

Frankel, A., Graydon-Baker, E., Neppi, C., Simmonds, T., Gustafson, M., & Gandhi, T. K. (2003). Patient safety: Patient safety leadership WalkRounds. *Joint Commission Journal on Quality and Safety.* Retrieved May 29, 2010, from http://www.ihi.org/ihi/search/searchresults.aspx? searchterm=walkrounds&searchtype=basic&Start+Search.x=0&Start+ Search.y=0

Garvin, D. A., & Roberto, M. A. (2001, October 15). What you don't know about making decisions. *Harvard Business School Working Knowledge.* Retrieved May 30, 2010, from http://hbswk.hbs.edu/item/2544.html

Gittel, J. H. (2003). *The Southwest Airlines Way: Using the power of relationships to achieve high performance.* New York: McGraw-Hill.

Griffin Hospital. (2009). *Griffin Hospital honored with tenth year on Fortune best companies to work for list.* Retrieved 20 March, 2011, from http:// www.griffinhealth.org/AboutUs/News/NewsReleases/tabid/362/ EntryId/203/Griffin-Hospital-Honored-with-Tenth-Year-on-FORTUNE-Best-Companies-to-Work-for-List.aspx

HealthGrades. (2010, March). *HealthGrades Seventh Annual Patient Safety in American Hospitals Study.* Retrieved January 30, 2011, from http://docs .google.com/viewer?a=v&q=cache:NaX9p1OSBkwJ:www.healthgrades .com/business/img/HealthGradesPatientSafetyRelease2010.pdf+ health+grades+seventh+annual+patient+safety+in+american&hl=en&gl =us&pid=bl&srcid=ADGEESi15tBRhtYRkxCBIw7Zpk26FFtHnojQgGrO fYlRld6B7TbSxmDj6Zx8SwUTQjqeKNNjr-vlOOiPwKbSvKxA4XNjUCb A7lekFNWvaAbiGcF0VlsWbUaF-QKP1MX0J4gFyi0xaGKz&sig=AHIEt bRytVqUxuN1Rp8jiqfwOC6XXemNDw

Institute for Healthcare Improvement. (n.d.) *IHI vision and values.* Retrieved June 5, 2010, from http://www.ihi.org/IHI/About/VisionValues/

Institute of Medicine. (2001). *Crossing the quality chasm: A new health system for the 21st century.* Retrieved January 1, 2011, from http://docs .google.com/viewer?a=v&q=cache:WYXMCzaAmCMJ:www.nap.edu/ html/quality_chasm/reportbrief.pdf+Crossing+the+Quality+Chasm:+ A+New+Health+System+for+the+21st+Century&hl=en&gl=us&pid=bl &srcid=ADGEESjRqFBCu7wyR8VhGHmalbi4-LdO4QxCNZyVZODcFV 7uzJ4NOaJbljwy1Hy9cm-lSyb3J4ux4CO7Zt3ur4UJ4BcXWNf4h0S1n BJOI8oH3S2-OkgrzS871M8APg_zWxiTRybipuil&sig=AHIEtbSetf7KJ4W MFrha10VYiFZkxtZwCg

Kaplan, S. (2008, June 15). *A PEP talk: What can you learn from successful CEO's?* Presented at the Convocation Ceremony University of Chicago Graduate School of Business.

Keppler Speakers. (n.d.). *About Gene Granz.* Retrieved March 3, 2011, from http://www.kepplerspeakers.com/speakers.aspx?name=Gene+Kranz

Keroack, M. A., Youngberg, B. J., Cerese, J. L., Krsek, C., Prellwitz, L. W., & Trevelyan, E. W. (2007). *Organizational factors associated with high performance in quality and safety in academic medical centers.* Retrieved May 30, 2010, from http://journals.lww.com/academicmedicine/Fulltext/2007/12000/ Organizational_Factors_Associated_with_High.14.aspx

Kreitner, R. (2007). *Management* (10th ed.). Canada: Houghton Mifflin Haurcourt Pub Co.

Laschinger, S., & Heather, K. (2006). The impact of nursing work environments on patient safety outcomes: The mediating role of burnout/engagement. *Journal of Nursing Administration, May 36*(5), 259–267.

Leider, R. J. (2004). *The Power of Purpose: Creating Meaning in Your Life and Work.* San Francisco: Bennet-Koehler.

Lundmark, V. A. (n.d.). *ARHQ: Chapter 46: Magnet environments for professional nursing practice.* [PDF electronic version] Retrieved May 22, 2010 from http://www.ahrq.gov/qual/nurseshdbk/

McFadden, K. L., Hengan, S. C., & Gowen, C. R. (2009). The patient safety chain: Transformational leadership's effect on patient safety culture, initiatives, and outcomes. *Journal of Operations Management.* Retrieved March 20, 2011, from http://docs.google.com/viewer?a=v&q=cache:LQ4d3c5q1NwJ :wweb.uta.edu/management/Dr.Casper/Fall10/BSAD6314/BSAD% 25206314-Student%2520Articles/Mediated%2520Multiple%2520Regre ssion/Mediation%2520Journal%2520of%2520Operations%2520Manag ement%2520(A.%2520Mehta).pdf+mcfadden+patient+safety+chain+m odel&hl=en&gl=us&pid=bl&srcid=ADGEESiNOcx1IdZib-yTknbhm7_ KIPCDi-3Ta6G3sU6ffxpAIu9RQljbyiFbDdI4-iDXRu8CGIEaUFuorVtkA

LTdJGO6CMR3njBq0MrLRJU69D1RI8y_Q3hn46gawHPTqeRIIyFIz6L9 &sig=AHIEtbQKceyGTu9Ed19Hw03M2QeI5FUfmw

Nelson, E. C., Batalden, P. B., Huber, T. P., Mohr, J. J., Godfrey, M. M., Headrick, L. A., et al. (2002). Microsystems in healthcare: Part 1. Learning from high-performing front-line clinical units. *The Joint Commission, 28*(9), pp. 472–493.

Peters, J., & Waterman, R. H. (1982). *In search of excellence: lessons from American's best run companies*. New York: Harper & Row.

Pink, D. H. (2009). *Drive: The surprising truth about what motivates us.* (Video) Retrieved May 24, 2010, from http://onecoolsitebloggingtips.com/ 2010/05/29/drive-the-surprising-truth-about-what-motivates-us/

Pittet, D. (2001). Improving adherence to hand hygiene practice: A multidisciplinary approach. *Emerging Infectious Diseases, (Special Issue) 7*(2), 234–240.

Pittet, D., Simon, A., Hugonnet, S., Pessoa-Silva, C. L., Sauvan, V., & Perneger, T. V. (2004). Hand hygiene among physicians: Performance, beliefs, and perceptions. *Annals of Internal Medicine.* Retrieved June 2, 2010, from http://www.psnet.ahrq.gov/resource.aspx?resourceID=1678

Planetree. (n.d.). *Planetree.* Retrieved May 1, 2011, from http://planetree. org; Retrieved February 20, 2011, from http://medicine.stanford.edu/ education/quality_improvement.html

Rami, C. (October 11, 2010) Defining effective leadership & effective decision making to build successful self-managed teams. Retrieved October 18, 2011 from http://www.innerwestlive.com.au/blog/2010/10/11/defining-effective-leadership-effective-decision-making-to-build-successful-self-managed-teams/

Rivera, R. L. (2010, March 15). Empowering people through self-managed teams. *Puerto Rico Daily Sun.* Retrieved May 30, 2010, from http://www .prdailysun.com/index.php?page=news.article&id=1268676242

Robert Wood Johnson Foundation. (2009). *New web site profiles 24 innovative nursing-driven models of health care delivery.* Retrieved January 11, 2011, from http://www.rwjf.org/reports/grr/057241.htm

Schnieder, J., Moromisato, D., Zemtra, B., Rizzi-Wagner, L., Rivero, N., Mason, W., et al. (2009). Hand hygiene adherence is influenced by the behavior of role models. *Pediatric Critical Care, 10*(3), pp. 360–363.

Senge, P. M. (1990). *The fifth discipline: The art & practice of the learning organization.* New York: Doubleday.

Smith, S.P., Flarey, D.L., (1999). *Process-Centered Healthcare Organizations.* Gaithersburg, Maryland: Aspen.

Southwest. (n.d.). *Southwest Airlines Fact Sheet.* Retrieved May 21, 2010, from http://www.southwest.com/about_swa/press/factsheet.html

Sredl, D., & Peng, N. H. (2010). CEO-CNE relationships: Building an evidence-base of chief nursing executive replacement costs. *International Journal of Medical Sciences.* Retrieved January 10, 2011, from http://www.medsci .org/v07p0160.htm

Vahey, D. C., Aiken, L. H., Sloane, D. M., Sean, P., & Vargas, D. (2004). Nurse burnout and patient satisfaction. *Medical Care.* Retrieved January 11, 2011, from http://journals.lww.com/lww-medicalcare/Abstract/2004/02001/ Nurse_Burnout_and_Patient_Satisfaction.8.asp

Zawacki, R. A., & Norman, C. A. (1994). Successful self-directed teams and planned change: A lot in common. *OD Practitioner. 33–38.*

10

Design at the Unit Level (Microsystem)

CLINICAL MICROSYSTEMS AND PATIENT SAFETY

Clinical microsystem is defined as a "small, interdependent group of people who work together regularly to provide care for specific groups of patients" (Institute for Healthcare Improvement [IHI], n.d.). These groups exist to serve a purpose (caring for specific populations) and are embedded in the overall organizational structures. They require information and administrative support to achieve their goals. Clinical microsystems involve nurses, physicians, other clinicians, and administrative support staff. For the microsystem to achieve its aim of caring for a specific population, the group shares work flow in clinical and business processes. They work within a shared informational environment that is embedded within the larger system of the organization. Microsystems, which provide the frontline interface for the delivery of care to patients, can be located anywhere in the health care system, from the intensive care units to primary care sites.

Research funded by the RWJF, conducted from 2000 to 2002 and published in June 2003 identified nine characteristics of high-performing clinical microsystems:

Leadership

Culture

Organizational support

Patient focus

Staff focus

Interdependence of the care team

Information and IT

Process improvement

Performance pattern

When applied to patient safety, the nine success characteristics might include

Leadership: The leadership sets the vision, values, and clear goals for the organization's patient safety program. The leadership role models the behaviors they expect of the staff. The leadership communicates effectively and frequently to reinforce the vision, values, and goals related to patient safety. This group aligns all formal and informal structures at the unit and the individual level to develop and sustain an effective patient safety culture.

Culture: The leadership greatly influences the patient safety culture of the organization. A just culture needs to be established along with role modeling of values related to patient safety. Leadership WalkRounds are established to assist with positive culture changes. Measurements of patient safety culture or climate, workplace culture, and quality of work life are all measured to actively seek opportunities for improvement.

Organizational support: The leadership provides the necessary resources and information to staff in order to develop a safer work environment and effective patient safety culture. Technology such as computerized physician order entry and bar codes are used with the aim of eliminating adverse events related to physician orders.

Patient focus: Patient-centered care is the model for care with emphasis on partnering with community resources. Patients are partners in care and in patient safety efforts. Full disclosure is done by the organization for any adverse events.

Staff focus: The value of human capital involves aligning staff with strategic goals. The right staff has the right competencies to utilize at the right time. Measurements are done for patient safety culture, quality of work life, and type of organizational culture with the aim to improve them.

Interdependence of care team: The care team is a high-performance team that shares a common purpose: to ensure that the six aims of safe, effective, timely, efficient, equitable, and patient-centered care are accomplished for every patient served. The team demonstrates competencies in communication, teamwork, and patient safety concepts.

Information and IT: The system incorporates the use of IT where feasible: computerized physician order entry, use of bar codes, and other tools that aim to greatly reduce and/or eliminate adverse events by forced functions or signaling the provider to warn him or her before taking the next action.

Process improvement: The NQF Safe Practices for Better Healthcare update contains 34 safe practices applicable to health care settings across the continuum of care with the aim of reducing the risk of harm to patients that results from processes, systems, and environments of care. These practices are evidence based.

Performance pattern: Key patient safety measures for preventable deaths and avoidable adverse events for patients and staff need to be measured and reported to the governing board and to staff with the aim to eliminate adverse events.

The Macolm Baldrige National Quality Award (MBNQA) has criteria within a model that the organization uses to perform its self-assessment and improvement. Foster, Johnson, Nelson, and Batalden (2007) compared the Malcolm Baldrige 14 health care criteria to the nine microsystem success characteristics noted above and found that they concurred, suggesting that these conceptual frameworks are congruent with each other. Further understanding of how the microsystem success characteristics and the Baldrige criteria relate to each other yields valuable information to better understand the Baldrige criteria and/or improve performance in a specific area needing improvement.

Mohr, Batalden, and Barach (2004) discussed the approach to improving safety within the clinical microsystem. They identified the clinical microsystem as an important level at which patient safety interventions should be focused. Because microsystems coexist with other microsystems across the organization, the cross microsystem relationships are essential to identifying opportunities for learning and improvement of quality and safety. In noting this, leadership also should make patient safety a priority and allow individual microsystems the authority to create innovative solutions for improvement.

Patient-Centered Care

The Commonwealth Fund authors Beach, Saha, and Cooper (2006) discussed patient centeredness and cultural competence as holding promise for quality improvement in providing care to individual patients, communities, and populations. They describe patient centeredness as originating in the late 1960s with several core features: understanding the patient as a unique person, exploring the experience of illness through the patient's viewpoint, searching for common ground in treatment modalities with the patient through the process of shared decision making, and building the physician–patient relationship. For its part, the Institute of Medicine (IOM) endorsed patient centeredness as one of the six aims for health system improvement in the 2001 *Crossing the Quality Chasm* report.

Attention to cultural competence, and the issues surrounding cultural competence, emerged in the medical literature in the early 1990s due to ongoing racial and ethnic disparities in health care. The goal of cultural competence is to increase health equity and reduce disparities by focusing on people of color as well as on all disadvantaged populations.

The primary goal of the patient centeredness movement was to provide individualized (customized) care and restore an emphasis on developing and sustaining personal relationships.

There was a recommendation that health care organizations and providers ensure that both patient centeredness and cultural competence are aligned in a manner to meet the needs of all patients.

Measurement pertaining to the degree of patient centeredness and cultural competence should be explored as part of any patient safety culture. According to Berwick (2009), "Patient centeredness is a dimension of health care quality in its own right, not just because of its connection with other desired aims, like safety and effectiveness. Its proper incorporation into new health care designs will involve some radical, unfamiliar, and disruptive shifts in control and power, out of the hands of those who give care and into the hands of those who receive it. Such a consumerist view of the quality of care, itself, has important differences from the more classical, professionally dominated definitions of 'quality.' New designs, like the so-called medical home, should incorporate that change.

Planetree is a nonprofit organization that provides education and information in a collaborative community of health care organizations, facilitating efforts to create patient-centered care in healing environments.

Since its founding in 1978, Planetree has continued to be a pioneer in personalizing, humanizing, and demystifying the health care experience for patients and their families. The Planetree model is committed to enhancing health care from the patient's perspective. It empowers patients and families through information and education and encourages "healing partnerships" with caregivers to support active participation. Through organizational transformation, the Planetree model creates healing environments in which patients can be active participants and caregivers are enabled to thrive.

The components of the Planetree model are as follows:

- *Human interactions/independence, dignity, and choice:* Through human beings caring for other human beings, a healing environment is created for patients, residents, families, and staff members. This includes providing personalized care for patients, residents, and their families as well as creating organizational cultures that support and nurture staff. A Planetree continuing care community offers a range of options that support an individual's autonomy, lifestyle, and interests. Residents direct their care, and consistent caregiving teams are assigned to strengthen relationships.
- *Importance of family, friends, and social support:* Social support is vital to good health without regard to the setting. Planetree encourages involvement of family and friends whenever possible, offers patient-directed visiting, including in the ICU and ER, and encourages the option of family presence during invasive procedures and resuscitation. The Care Partner Program promotes a heightened level of family participation while patients are hospitalized and at home after discharge. Families are encouraged to stay overnight whenever possible. Beyond the human family, pet therapy can elevate mood, lower blood pressure, and enhance social interaction.
- *Patient/resident education and community access to information:* Illness is seen as an educational and potentially transformational opportunity. An open chart policy encourages patients to read their medical records. Patients may write in Patient's Progress Notes in their medical record and may participate in a self-medication program enabling them to keep medications at the bedside. Collaborative care conferences, patient pathways, and a variety of educational resources provide patients and residents with information and skills to actively participate in their care as well as maximize their physical and psychological well-being. Patient and family libraries along with Internet access are available, and Planetree Health Resource Centers are open to the community and offer health and medical information on a wide range of topics.
- *Healing environment: architecture and interior design:* The physical environment is vital to healing and well-being. Each hospital and

continuing care community is designed to incorporate the comforts of home, clearly valuing humans, not just technology. By removing architectural barriers, the design encourages patient and family involvement. An awareness of the symbolic messages communicated by the design is an essential part of planning. Spaces are provided for both solitude and social activities, including libraries, kitchens, lounges, activity rooms, chapels, gardens, and overnight accommodation for families.

- *Nutritional and nurturing aspects of food:* Nutrition is integral to healing, essential not only for good health but also as a source of pleasure, comfort, and familiarity. A flexible dining program that encourages fellowship is particularly relevant in continuing care settings. Health care organizations become role models for delicious, healthy eating, with kitchens available throughout the facility to encourage families to bring the patient's favorite food from home or prepare meals for themselves. Volunteers bake breads, muffins, and cookies to provide "aromatherapy" and to create a nurturing environment.

- *Arts program/meaningful activities and entertainment:* Planetree recognizes that people need opportunities for camaraderie, laughter, and creativity, and a variety of classes, events, music, storytellers, clowns, and funny movies create an atmosphere of serenity and playfulness. Artwork in patient rooms, treatment areas, and residential spaces adds to the ambiance. Art carts enable patients to select the artwork of their choice. Volunteers work with patients and residents who would like to create their own art, whereas artists, musicians, poets and storytellers from the local community help to expand the boundaries of the health care facility. In continuing care settings, staff plans and participates in activities to build fellowship.

- *Spirituality and diversity:* Planetree recognizes the vital role of spirituality in healing the whole person. Supporting patients, residents, families, and staff in connecting with their own inner resources enhances the healing environment. Chapels, gardens, labyrinths, and meditation rooms provide opportunities for reflection and prayer. Chaplains are seen as vital members of the health care team.

- *Importance of human touch:* Touch reduces anxiety, pain, and stress benefiting patients, residents, families, and caregivers. Training programs for staff and family caregivers and volunteers to learn hand and foot rubs and internship programs for massage therapists keep costs minimal.

- *Integrative therapies/paths to well-being:* Expand the choices offered to patients and residents beyond western scientific care. Aromatherapy, acupuncture, and Reiki are examples of expanded options offered in addition to clinical modalities of care. To meet growing consumer demand for complementary therapies, Planetree affiliates have instituted heart disease reversal programs, guided imagery, therapeutic touch, acupuncture, Tai Chi, and yoga. Aromatherapy's calming effect on agitated patients is useful to augment pain management modalities and decrease anxiety. Exercise facilities customized for seniors offer programs to improve strength, balance, and fitness. Wellness programs focus on prevention and chronic disease management.

■ *Healthy communities/enhancement of life's journey:* Working with schools, senior citizen centers, churches, and other community partners, hospitals are redefining health care to include the health and wellness of the larger community. Choosing environmentally friendly cleaning products and sponsoring "kid's camps," walking clubs, and community gardens expands the role of hospitals from treating illness to promoting wellness. Continuing care communities offer opportunities for personal growth, self-expression, and fulfillment of individual dreams. Life Stories programs capture milestones in a resident's life and enable caregivers to see a whole person, nurturing a bond with residents. (Used with permission of Planetree)

Planetree has experienced superior performance on the Hospital Consumer Assessment of Healthcare Provider and Systems (HCAHPS).

Isacc, Zaslavsky, Cleary, and Landon (2010) looked at the degree to which patient experiences with hospital care were related to other measures of hospital quality and safety using service-line specific data in 927 hospitals in a national study. There were consistent relationships between patient experiences and technical quality as measured by measures used in the Hospital Quality Alliance programand complication rates as measured by the AHRQ Patient Safety Indicators. Two overall measures of hospital performance, the overall rating of the hospital and willingness to recommend the hospital had strong relationships with better technical performance in processes of care related to pneumonia, CHF, myocardial infarction, and for surgical care. Better patient experiences in all HCAHPS domains were also associated with lower decubitus ulcer rates. Other complications such as infections due to medical care were strongly related to patient experiences in specific domains, such as whether the hospital environment was clean and quiet and whether the staff was communicative and responsive.

Recently, Planetree received grant money from the Commonwealth fund for a 6-month project to develop a refined set of designation criteria with objective outcome metrics by which patient centeredness across continuing care settings can be evaluated. The findings of this project are planned to be widely disseminated and the instrument may be viable for endorsement by the NQF.

Culture at the Unit Level and Patient Safety

Culture is the key driver for implementing an effective patient safety program. Changing organizational cultures is not an easy task; it requires profound change efforts. When patient safety programs focus only on the tasks that require implementation, however, little progress is made. Nurses, who play a major role in patient safety ever caring for patients on the front line, require a redesigned system that is conducive to safe and professional practice. The Magnet program, for example, offers a model for a system's framework that can enhance safe and professional practice at the bedside.

However, the American Nurses Credentialing Center (ANCC)'s website shows that only 382 facilities have attained Magnet status out of 5,815 hospitals in the United States, a small, if still growing, number of hospitals indeed.

According to Senge (1999), profound change requires organizational change that combines inner shifts in staff values, aspirations and resulting behaviors which result in outer shifts in processes, strategies, practices, and, of course, systems. This process, building the capacity for ongoing change, also requires continuous learning and dialogue. It means that staff must be provided the opportunity to interact with each other in a meaningful way that promotes dialogue, reflection, and thinking.

Example 1: You walk into a hospital clinic. It has warm colors on the walls and the patients are sitting on chairs, patiently waiting for their appointment. There is a centralized nursing station that serves as a reception area, nurses are dressed in white uniforms, and there are identifiable intersections in tasks. There is a reception area for greeting patients and admitting them into the system, waiting areas for patients and families to sit in, and clinic exam rooms. The noise level mixes the conversations of patients and nurses, and the hustle in the hallways involves physicians, technicians, and nurses. Patients are being escorted to and from exam rooms. There is a certain assembly-line feel to it. Staff use jargon when assisting patients and telling them where to go for diagnostics: MRI, pre-op admin clinic, working up patients prior to surgery, and so on.

Example 2: Next, you walk into the intensive care unit. There are no patients or family members sitting in chairs; the patients in bed are on ventilators, attached to all kinds of tubes. The nurses are dressed in various colors of scrub suits.

Tubes are visibly seen attached to machines for monitoring and maintaining physiologic functions such as blood pressure, oxygen levels, and nutritional support.

The noise level consists of alarms going off intermittently, the whirr and hum of machines, and the spoken technical jargon from staff.

The physicians and nurses are talking in a language that is specialized to their area. "Mr. Smith has multifocal PVCs (premature ventricular contractions) and PCWPs (pulmonary capillary wedge pressures) are high. Mr. Smith is hypotensive, tachycardiac, and is receiving titrating IV medications to increase urine output and blood pressure."

There are observable clusters of care in the intensive care unit. As the physicians round with the nurses and ancillary staff, the language of each specialty is heard. There is an urgency and quickness of pace. Emergent care interrupts the rounds, and the attending physician, residents, and nurses rush to one of the bedside of a patient who has "coded."

Example 3: Operating rooms consist of dominant hierarchies of multiple surgeons in multiple specialties and each surgery requires teamwork that is complex, fast-paced, with little or no margin for error.

You walk into an operating room and again the language is different; medical jargon specific to the operating room. The personalities at work in the operating room are also very different than those in the outpatient clinic area or in the intensive care area.

The outpatient clinic area is focused on interpersonal and diagnostic skills; the intensive care area is focused on stabilizing critical physiologic parameters; and the operating room staff is focused on the technical skills and competencies required to get the patient safely through operative procedures.

The operating room has increased technology usage, and tight interdependencies of team tasks are required. For example, the right instrument has to be used for the right task, at the right time, using the right technique, and each task performed must have high reliability. The operating room and Ic are considered high-risk areas due to the complexity and coordination of care required among the various groups of staff for consistent outcomes to be achieved.

Just as different units within a health care organization have variation in cultures, so do various groups of staff. Physicians are responsible for setting a working atmosphere on patient care units, and this affects nurses along with ancillary staff.

The term "culture" refers to the values and beliefs that are shared within an organization. Culture is dynamic. Culture is something with a past, living in the present, and influencing the future. Patient safety culture is a subset of the organizational culture. Wilbert (2001) described a safety culture as one that comprises at least three analytical levels, from the deep layer of often unconscious basic assumptions and orientations, progressing to shared values and norms, then to directly observable behavior patterns. Fleming (2005) reported that the Advisory Committee on the Safety of Nuclear Installations (ACSNI) defined patient safety culture in 1993 as "the product of individual and group values, attitudes, perceptions, competencies, and patterns of behavior that determine the commitment to, and proficiency of, an organization's health and safety management." Another way of saying this is that safety culture is an organization's collective beliefs and values in which priority is placed on patient safety by everyone, from the hospital administrator to the janitor. A patient safety culture reflects the extent that everyone commits to personal responsibility and actions that communicate safety concerns.

According to the IOM, "the biggest challenge to moving toward a safer health system is changing the culture from one of blaming individuals for errors to one in which errors are treated not as personal failures, but as opportunities to improve the system and prevent harm."

AHRQ offers a free toolkit that measures the following dimensions in patient safety culture:

Communication openness

Feedback and communication about error

Frequency of events reported

Hospital handoffs and transitions

Hospital management support for patient safety

Nonpunitive response to error

Organizational learning–continuous improvement

Overall perceptions of safety

Staffing

Supervisor or manager expectations and actions promoting patient safety

Teamwork across hospital units

Teamwork within units

The toolkit can be accessed at www.ahrq.gov/qual/patientsafety culture/hospsurvindex.htm#Toolkit

Agency for Healthcare Research and Quality (AHRQ) (2009) results from Hospital Survey on Patient Safety Culture consisted of 395 hospitals that participated in previous survey reports along with 104 hospitals submitting data for the first time and 123 hospitals submitting data from re-administering the survey and replacing the old results with the updated survey results. Average response rate per hospital was 52 percent. Nearly 200,000 categories of hospital staff responded to the survey.

The two areas that emerged as organizational strengths related to teamwork within units (79 percent positive response) and self-scores for patient safety grade with 73 percent grading their work area or unit grade as A—Excellent (25 percent), and B—Very good (48 percent).

Areas with potential for improvement for most hospitals:

Nonpunitive response to error: This was cited as an area for improvement within most hospitals. Only 44 percent of staff felt that their mistakes and event reports were not held against them or maintained in personnel files.

Handoffs and transitions: This area received only a positive 44 percent for transferring patient information with patients across hospital units and shift changes.

Number of events reported: Approximately 50 percent, on average, of the hospitals reported no events in their hospital over the past 12 months.

Nonteaching hospitals: Nonteaching hospitals reported the highest positive scores for teamwork across units and handoffs and transitions.

Government hospitals: Government hospitals were more positive than nongovernment hospitals for handoffs and transitions (6 percent more positive).

There is wide variation among subcultures, groups, and categories of workers.

Culture can be thought of as being similar to a large body of water that looks calm at the surface but has numerous currents and eddies at varying levels underneath the surface. It is beneath the surface that the real story of the culture of various departments, groups, and subgroups is found.

Two dominant professional cultures relate to physicians and nurses. The physician culture also has subcultures and groups within it, as does nursing.

For example, one could argue that the surgeon culture is different than the internal medicine group culture. One could also argue that an Ic nurse group may have a different culture than nurses who work in rehabilitation or palliative care.

Dickey, Daminao, and Ungerleider (2003) recalled the story of the events that happened at Duke University where incompatible lungs were transplanted into a teenage girl leading to her eventual death. They stated that the hierarchic structure created an environment where the surgeon accepted full responsibility for the mistake, rather than one in which the shortcomings of the system would be examined. This example reflected how culture feeds the news media and reinforces the public's worst fears regarding the health care system. They stated that surgeons were trained to be the "captain of the ship" and own the responsibility for care. Surgeons frequently lack the skills that come from collaborative teamwork and they tend to view mistakes as unacceptable. Health care organizations frequently create elaborate strategic goals, write the quality and patient safety plan, and a few years later wonder what went wrong.

Patient Safety Culture Versus Patient Safety Climate

The saying of "culture eats strategy for breakfast" is a common one. For sure, culture will nibble at strategy persistently until the strategy exists no more.

Measurement of patient safety culture is a relatively new Joint Commission requirement and provides only a foundation on which to anchor future improvement efforts.

The Committee on Quality of Healthcare in America, IOM report *To Err Is Human: Building a Safer Health System* (2000) recommended that health care organizations "must develop a culture of safety such that an organization's care processes and workforce are focused on improving the reliability and safety of care for patients." This requires the dedication and commitment of the organization's top leadership.

Anyone who works in quality knows that aggregation of information is important to know system progress; however, it is only through stratification that we begin to understand and take the appropriate actions to reduce variability and improve overall performance. This is the key difference between an organization's patient safety *culture* and patient safety *climate*.

Patient safety climate was described by Dr. Sexton in his interview with AHRQ (n.d.-a) as the extent to which the frontline caregivers possess a genuine and proactive commitment to patient safety within a specific patient care area. There is a great deal of variation across hospital units in patient safety culture. The Ic may have a very good patient safety climate whereas the general medical floor may have a poor one.

Patient safety climate has different attributes than a patient safety culture even though sometimes these terms are used interchangeably. A patient safety climate deals with perceptions of staff at selected areas within a health care organization to situational and environmental factors at a given point in time. For example, an Ic may have a very different patient safety climate than the clinic setting.

Patient safety culture measures the health care organization's collective attitudes, values, and patterns of behaviors for shared perceptions of the importance of patient safety. This is characterized by trust of staff to disclose errors and continuously learn from them.

Both accreditation and patient safety are driven by the organizational culture. The Joint Commission requires that the leadership at accredited organizations regularly evaluate the culture of safety and quality. This evaluation must use valid and reliable tools.

According to AHRQ's Patient Safety Network (n.d.-b), a safety culture has key components similar to those in high-reliability organizations such as nuclear power plants, which consistently minimize adverse events. These organizations are also complex systems where hazardous work is carried out.

The key features are:

There is an acknowledgement of the high-risk nature of the work carried out on a daily basis along with the determination to achieve consistent safe operations.

There is a blame-free environment and individuals are able to report errors or near misses without fear of reprimand or punishment.

There is encouragement for collaboration across ranks and disciplines to find solutions to patient safety problems.

There is a commitment from the organization to provide resources to address safety concerns.

Two patient safety surveys discussed earlier in the chapter that have been validated are the AHRQ's Patient Safety Culture Survey and the Safety Attitudes Questionnaire. The AHRQ provides comparative results for the Patient Safety Culture Survey and the toolkit is available online at www.ahrq.gov/qual/patientsafetyculture/hospsurvindex.htm.

The Safety Attitudes Questionnaire has been administered to over 10,000 providers in 203 clinical areas and in three countries. It measures domains for provider attitudes that include teamwork climate, safety climate, perceptions of management, job satisfaction, working conditions, and stress recognition (Sexton et al., 2006).

Why is it important to measure safety attitudes at the unit level? It is because a health care organization has wide variation in cultures at the unit levels. Think of the nature and complexity of the Ic versus the clinic.

The patient population is different, the tasks demanded in the workload are different, the arrangement of the teams required to provide care to the patient are also different, and the communication patterns are different. It is not surprising that the cultures that develop over time will also be different.

Nurse Hierarchy Importance in Change Efforts

A study by Kalish and Begeny (2007) reported results from two geographically separate hospitals involving a total of 578 nurses using the "I Opt" instrument that measures information processing preferences results. The aim of this research was to study the ability of nurses at the unit level to "accept, adopt and sponsor change in an era of high volatility in health care."

The "I Opt" tool is based on the idea that the kind of information that is sought and accepted from the environment hinders or enhances certain types of behaviors. So, for example, if a person does not pay attention to details, then the person will not be precise in his or her responses. There are four information-processing styles:

Reactive Stimulator (RS): This pattern tends to accept change but the risk is in moving too fast. This is called a performer pattern.

Hypothetical Analyzer (HA): The focus is on doing things right. The risk relates to over-caution with potential hesitance to fully commit to a change initiative. This is named a conservator style.

Relational Innovator (RI): Deliberate, detail-oriented, and precise, combined with reacting quickly to novel and unexpected ideas. This is called a split style. Responses tend to be split between very different approaches.

Logical Processer (LP): Action-oriented with a high value on doing things "right." The ability to see the complexity in situations tends to make the person a bit skeptical of the change effort or the ultimate success of the change effort.

Kalish and Begeny's findings included the following:

Nurses most closely resembled customer service personnel with no significant difference across all four "I Opt" strategic styles between nurses and customer service personnel. Customer service typically involves a person answering client questions by referring to approved information sources.

Nurses demonstrated significant differences among all four "I Opt" strategic styles when compared with engineers, scientists, and corporate managers. Nurses scored lower in the unpatterned input strategies of RI (ideas) and RS (decisive action). These two strategic styles are able to initiate and accommodate change without much difficulty.

Nurses in intensive care and psychiatric areas were more idea-oriented (RI) than other specialties. The authors stated these areas encounter experiences that do not yield to standardized approaches, where surgical was significantly lower in spontaneous decisive action (RS). The authors stated that in areas such as the operating room, nurses have little autonomy for independent nursing action.

Nurses were the least able to initiate and accept change among the functions reviewed. Their favored information processing strategy relied on certainty, a step-by-step operational knowledge.

Nurse managers had much higher levels of ideas (RI) and decisive actions (RS) than the staff nurses from all specialties. This means that nurse managers think differently from staff nurses, and nurse managers need to be taught how to lead others who think differently than they do.

Nurse aides obtained significantly higher scores for disciplined action than the registered nurses did. This was interpreted as meaning that the registered nurses, who are reluctant to change, would be enhanced by the nurse aides who support them.

Unit secretaries were more committed to discipline action than were the registered nurses. This adds another layer of unit resistance to change that regularly interacts and influences the registered nurses.

Licensed practical nurses were also significantly more committed to disciplined action than were the registered nurses, which adds yet another layer of change resistance below the level of the registered nurse.

The authors concluded that the registered nurse at the unit level sits on another layer of unit personnel even more resistant to change than they are, and since these roles continually interact with the registered nurse, they are positioned to make the registered nurses' basic resistance to change even worse.

The recommendations from this study were for executives to remember that addressing just the registered nurses is not sufficient; change efforts must target the support staff as well, a requirement that will likely make a difficult job even more difficult.

Ethics on the Front Line of Care

Nurses on the front line experience numerous situations where they face moral questions of what is right and wrong. According to Lachman (2006), an ethical dilemma involves a problem with choices that seem or are equally unfavorable. ANA has a Code of Ethics for Nurses, which identifies the ethical obligations for all nurses. The ANA Code of Ethics for Nurses (American Nurses Association [ANA], 2001) provides the framework for ethical decision making and reinforces nursing as a profession. The nurse's primary commitment is always to the patient, and the nurse consistently serves as the patient's advocate to protect the health, safety, and rights of the patient. Considering this in the context of the current patient safety environment, it is essential for nurses to have a voice that is heard and supported when he or she reports medical errors and/or bad behavior that prevent collaboration and cooperation at the frontline level.

Bad Behavior

Most nurses have experienced conflict with other health care professionals and conflict within their own profession as well. I remember being a new graduate and taking a job in an Ic in a large teaching hospital. I was overwhelmed with trying to learn new procedures, new assessments, new knowledge pertaining to the care of complex, critically ill patients, and new interactions with peers, physicians, and other health care professionals.

The experienced nurses varied in their kindness: some were very willing to teach and share their knowledge; others would share their knowledge and belittle you while they were doing it; and few others would not share any knowledge and berate you for asking them a question. It was a tough, competitive environment with a high turnover rate.

The Joint Commission (2008) issued a *Sentinel Event Alert* to stop bad behavior, specifically rude language and hostile behavior because "these behaviors can foster medical errors, contribute to poor patient satisfaction, to preventable adverse outcomes, increase the cost of care, and cause qualified clinicians, administrators, and managers to seek new positions in more professional environments."

The Joint Commission acknowledged that there has been a long history of tolerance and indifference to disruptive behaviors and that many of these events go unreported and therefore are not handled by anyone. They cited an ACPE survey where respondents reported that approximately 40 percent of the time, "physicians in my organization who generate high amounts of revenue are treated more leniently when it comes to behavior problems than those who bring in less revenue."

Physicians' and nurses' cultures need to change from dysfunctional to a patient safety culture starting with their professional education. This is where they are taught the basics when they are learning their new work competencies. The Joint Commission implemented two new standards that were effective in January 2009:

The hospital or organization has a code of conduct that defines acceptable and disruptive and inappropriate behaviors.

Leaders create and implement a process for managing disruptive and inappropriate behaviors.

The ANA (2010) published a paper written by Rowell on lateral violence known as "nurse against nurse." Reasons for lateral violence described were related to role issues, oppressed group issues, gender issues, and self-esteem issues.

Role issues: Nurses have role issues with physicians who are taught clinical autonomy combined with a "captain of the ship" mentality. Nurses are taught to work in teams. Nurses wish to work in a collaborative fashion; physicians tend to wish to work in a hierarchical fashion. Also, nurses have diverse roles within their own profession with variation in cultures. Role issues arise between levels of staff, between different categories of staff, and within different competency levels of staff.

Oppressed group issues: This type of behavior occurs when one group feels it has been excluded from the power structure. When this occurs, abuse may occur to peers and to health care workers of lesser status.

Gender issues: Nurses do not see themselves as equals to physicians in power; they have been socialized to be the server (and nurturer). When nurses have feelings related to gender issues, it leads to frustration, anger, and/or fear and these feelings can be displaced laterally or downward.

Self-esteem issues: The research indicates that what is experienced by interactions during the nurses training shapes his or her professional image later, and self-esteem is a major consideration within all of the approaches to lateral violence.

Entitlement (potential issue): When a person feels entitled to certain privileges that their peer group is not granted he/she may be a target of lateral violence.

Cooper et al. (2009) reported a nonexperimental descriptive study where 636 participants (nursing students) completed a Bullying in Nursing Education Questionnaire (BNEQ). They reported that 56 percent of bullying behaviors were experienced from their classmates. The most frequent bullying behaviors included cursing, swearing, inappropriate behaviors, belittling, or humiliating. The most frequent response by the student to the bullying behavior was "did nothing."

The researchers concluded that there need to be strategies at the university level that include zero tolerance policies and education and training for students and faculty, along with health care agency employees.

Halverson (2010) reported on some interesting facts about bullying in the workplace. She reported the ISMP study where 88 percent of the medical practitioners surveyed experienced condescending language or voice intonation, 87 percent experienced impatience with questions asked, 79 percent dealt with a reluctance or a refusal to answer questions, 48 percent experienced strong, verbal abuse, and 43 percent experienced actual threatening of body language. Four percent actually experienced physical abuse.

Halverson also reported that bullies are very expensive for organizations to maintain. According to her reports, conservative estimates and prevalent data indicate that "bullying medical practitioners cost organizations over a million dollars per 50 employees per year in turnover costs alone."

The Workplace Bullying Institute (WBI) shared the results of its 2010 workplace bullying survey. There were two surveys conducted, one with several items and 4,210 respondents and one single-item survey with 2,092 respondents. Each sample was a representative sample of all American adults in August 2010. The major findings:

Thirty-five percent of workers have experienced bullying firsthand.

The majority of bullies are men (62 percent); 58 percent of the targets are women.

Women bullies target women in 80 percent of the cases.

Thirty-five percent of the U.S. workforce, or approximately 53.5 million Americans, report being bullied at work. Although half of all Americans have experienced bullying directly, 50 percent report that they have never experienced it or witnessed it.

What is even more discouraging is that the top level may perceive the bully as a good employee. According to O'Brien (2000), this is because the three most frequent bullying tactics used by bosses were reported as (1) blame for errors, (2) unreasonable job demands, and (3) criticism of ability.

The health care environment should be one in which workers interact with others with "respect for person" as the basis for all communications. Better communication skills need to be acquired at all levels.

This involves training the physicians and nurses the right time, the right way, to provide the right knowledge, skills, and attitudes to care for patients in the 21st century.

It does not stop there. All health care workers, starting from top level administrators to the janitors, need to have training on patient safety concepts and communication techniques so that everyone on the team has common values in regard to respect for person, when communicating their positions on providing patient care.

Disclosure at the Unit Level

Patients trust health care professionals to do the right thing. There is a relationship of trust. When health care providers are not fully honest with patients and families, it harms both patient and public trust. Once trust is lost, it is very difficult to regain. The Joint Commission implemented the requirement for all hospitals to disclose to patients all unexpected outcomes of care.

Example 1: A surgeon makes a misdiagnosis and fails to intervene for appendicitis; the patient's appendix ruptures and he experiences an extended hospital stay and recovery period. The surgeon does not want to disclose the mistake to the patient because no real harm was done and the patient will not detect the error.

Example 2: A medical intern makes a mistake and orders 10 times the normal dose of an antibiotic, which then causes the patient to suffer extensive liver damage. The intern discloses the error to the patient but does not disclose his responsibility in the error.

Witman, Park, and Hardin (1996) reported the results from a survey where 98 percent of internal medicine patients expressed their wishes that there be some acknowledgment of even minor errors that might occur to them. For both moderate and severe mistakes, patients were significantly more likely to consider filing a medical-legal suit if the physician did not disclose the error to them. The authors concluded with reinforcing the critical importance of maintaining open communication between patients and physicians.

In a survey in 2002 by Lam, Studdert, Bohmer, Berwick, and Brennan, stratified random sampling was done to select 500 hospitals from the AHA's database of 1,218 medical/surgical hospitals with greater than 200 beds. The response rate for the survey was 54 percent. The results were as follows:

Approximately 33 percent of the hospitals had board-approved disclosure policies in place, and 54 percent reported that it was routine practice to tell patients and their families when a patient had been harmed, and another 44 percent stated they disclosed at least some of the time. Only five respondents stated their hospital did not disclose harms.

When there was serious injury or death, 65 percent of the hospitals reported always disclosing these events to patients and families.

The forms that disclosure took in these hospitals had the common elements of an explanation, an undertaking to look into the incident and see what happened, and an apology with an acknowledgment of harm. However, relatively few respondents reported that the typical disclosure included acknowledging responsibility for the harm or that sharing of investigation results occurred with the patients and families.

Fear of medical malpractice litigation was the most cited institutional barrier to developing and to implementing disclosure policies, followed by staff opposition.

The authors concluded that at least 98 percent of the hospitals disclosed medical harm to patients at least some of the time, and 80 percent have disclosure policies in place or under development; however, there was still marked variation in the types of harm that hospitals were prepared to disclose and how they handled such disclosures.

Gallagher et al. (2006) reported on a survey mailed to 2,637 medical and surgical physicians in the United States. The physicians received one of four scenarios outlining serious errors that varied by medical and surgical scenarios and how obvious the error would be to the patient if not disclosed.

The results reported demonstrated a wide variation regarding what information the respondents would disclose, with 51 percent of the respondents who received the more apparent error explicitly mentioning the error, whereas only 32 percent mentioned the error when they received the less apparent error. Also, medical specialists had a higher percentage of explicitly mentioning the error: 58 percent compared to 19 percent with their surgical counterparts.

The researchers concluded that more disclosure standards and training are necessary to meet public expectations and also to enhance professional responsibility when errors are made.

Fein et al. (2005) described a conceptual model for disclosure of medical errors that included the following elements:

The institutional culture: Institutional culture involves the perceptions by staff on the error tolerance and supportive infrastructure. There are various subcultures within the institutional culture. For example, if the institutional culture is tolerant but the nursing culture is not, or if the nursing culture is tolerant but one of the nurse managers is not, it affects disclosure.

Provider factors: There are many provider factors affecting the degree and type of disclosure: fear of malpractice, loss of reputation, loss of job, loss of positive relationship with the patient, perceived professional responsibility, type of medical training, lack of confidence in disclosure skills, and personal discomfort associated with disclosure.

Error factors: The degree of harm that actually occurred to the patient and if the patient will be likely to be aware of the error contribute to the likelihood that full disclosure will take place.

Nondisclosure of medical mistakes: Nondisclosure prevents learning from occurring and also erodes patient and public trust in the health care system.

CBC News (2009) reported that when Montreal Jewish Hospital in Montreal, Canada implemented a full disclosure policy regarding medical mistakes made during patient care, they experienced a 50 percent drop in their adverse incidents over the past 3 years.

Hospital staff are being encouraged to report and learn from the incident.

The American Society for Healthcare Risk Management of the AHA (American Society for Healthcare Risk Management [ASHRM], 2003a, 2003b) published a three-part series on disclosure. In the first report, the following models of disclosure were discussed:

One-person model: The provider or other person designated (e.g., risk manager) goes in alone and discloses the event to the patient and family. The benefits of this involve having a designated person who can be trained and acquire the communication skills necessary for effective disclosure. The drawbacks discussed related to having no room for any shared responsibility or disseminating the philosophy of disclosure throughout the organization. This type of model may fit best in a small organization.

Team model: A select group of staff from the various services are trained. This group then coaches physicians/clinicians and pairs up with them when disclosure is done. The benefits for this approach are, again, that the organization should have consistency in the disclosure information that the patient receives. The drawback for this disclosure model relates to health care staff being diverted from their normal duties to participate as a coach in a disclosure discussion. This type of model may fit best in a small–medium size organization.

Trainer model: The organization invests in a comprehensive training program for a large group of physicians and other staff. The trained individuals then train and receive a reward for training a set number of staff each year. The trainers become both mentors and role models. The benefits for this model included the organization's capacity to disseminate the philosophy and skill set for disclosure throughout the organization. The drawbacks involve the consistency and quality control of the skill set along with distribution of responsibility to ensure that trainers are training at the level expected. This model may fit best in large- to medium-sized organizations that are spread out geographically.

Time coaching model: The individual practitioner at the event discloses what is known at that time. In this model, the disclosure may be made by a nurse, attending physician, or other practitioner with whom the patient has a relationship. The benefits of this model are simplicity and directness. The responsibility for disclosure is at the point of care. The drawbacks involve the skill level of the individual who does the disclosure at the point of care. Where communication skills are effective, this is felt to be the ideal model; however, the success is dependent on the communication skills of the person who is disclosing the event. This model may fit best in organizations that have grown and matured in their patient safety culture.

ASHRM concluded their first paper with recommendations that health care organizations move from disclosure to communication and involve integrating the concept of open communication into all aspects of the health care environment. This will involve the patient as a partner and also involve other members of the health care team working together to create safe processes.

Part II of the ASHRM (2003a, 2003b) disclosure series provided a framework for developing an organizational policy for effective patient communication. The objective was written for this as "Hospital X believes that patients are entitled to information about the outcomes of diagnostic tests, medical treatment, and surgical intervention."

Hospital X and its providers recognize the importance of maintaining good communication with patients and, when appropriate, their family by providing information that fosters informed decision making. Definitions for the policy included "Adverse event error or unanticipated event, near miss, Sentinel event, significant adverse event, disclosure, Patient Safety Committee and/or Patient Safety Officer, informed consent, primary caregiver, outcome, patient care or treatment plan."

The criteria for identifying the types of events that warrant disclosure were advised to be brief and included generalized language to allow for various types of events to be included.

Roles and responsibilities related to disclosure are described. Who will be responsible to provide the disclosure, and what does the organization wish to say to the patient and family on a consistent basis? There needs to be accommodation for any special communication needs the patient might have, any support services available, steps for any follow-up conversations, and documentation of the conversation in the medical record. Resolution steps for any stage of conflict, ranging from pastoral care to calling security for aggressiveness, should be addressed via the policy. There should be a section that addresses the rare circumstance where disclosure may not be appropriate and the steps to take when this occurs. The plan should include dates when the policy will be reviewed again and when the policy was implemented.

Polices need to adapt to special populations and care settings. All staff need to be educated on the policy and should know their role. The goal of an effective communication plan, as ASHRM puts it, is "Safe and trusted health care."

Part III of the ASHRM (2004) disclosure series described what would work even better than disclosure. In this series, ASHRM emphasized that disclosure was an ethical obligation, not just a regulatory requirement, and that disclosure, when done properly, can potentially lessen the frequency and severity of litigation. Within this series, a skills-based model for disclosure is presented. This model involves a solid presentation to the patient of the facts that are known at the time of the disclosure, with no more than two people, one of which is the physician.

The complete monograph series on disclosure from ASHRM can be accessed at the Premier website at www.premierinc.com/quality/tools-services/safety/topics/patient_safety/sample-policies.jsp.

Also, IHI has an example of a disclosure policy at www.ihi.org/IHI/Topics/PatientSafety/SafetyGeneral/Tools/SeriousEvent DisclosurePolicyWentworthDouglass.htm.

When patients are harmed, full disclosure needs to be done skillfully and compassionately as soon as possible after the event. Communication skills are key to ensuring success. The other aspect of disclosure relates to the health care professional acknowledging that an error has been made. When there is a culture of blame within the organization, health care professionals are reluctant to report errors. Disclosure involves trust that the reporting of the error will be handled fairly by the leaders.

Honest mistakes should never be punished and reckless behaviors should never be tolerated. There is an ethical duty to disclose medical errors at the provider level and at the administrative level to handle disclosure of medical errors by using "just culture" principles.

There needs to be clarity on what constitutes a medical error so that health care professionals know what is expected to be reported.

When adverse events occur, there needs to be a support system for the person who committed the honest mistake. Staff join the health care profession to help people, not harm them. They deserve to have a support system to be there for them when needed. When staff feel supported, they are less likely to play the blame game where the organization, the staff, and the patient lose. The organization loses because there is a high likelihood that future events will not get reported; the individual loses because there might be increased stress and a higher likelihood for making another error in the future. The patient loses because the medical error might be repeated.

Physician Decisions and Medical Error

Baum (n.d.) advocated that there needs to be support to translate the best current science into individual clinical practice decisions. Health care decisions that are unsupported by the best science increase the chance of errors and need to be eliminated. There needs to be an effort to reduce the variation in clinical practice when that variation deviates from good scientific evidence.

Groopman (2007) argued that statistics deal with averages, and patients are not averages; patients are individuals. According to Groopman, the experts recently concluded that the majority of errors are not technical mistakes but are due to flaws in physician thinking. "In one study of misdiagnoses that cause serious harm to patients, some 80 percent could be accounted for by a cascade of cognitive errors." He went on to state that physicians make errors 15 percent of the time when they make a diagnosis.

Graber, Franklin, and Gordon (2005) reviewed 100 cases of diagnostic error; 90 cases involved injury, which included 33 deaths. The underlying contributions to error fell into the categories of no fault, system-related, and cognitive. Only seven cases reflected no-fault errors alone. For the remaining 93 cases, 548 different system-related or cognitive factors were identified. The system-related factors contributed to diagnostic error in 65 percent of the cases and cognitive factors in 74 percent of the cases.

The most common system-related factors involved problems with policies and procedures, processes that were inefficient, teamwork that was inefficient, or communication that was inefficient. The cognitive problem that was the most common involved faulty synthesis. The single most common cause was the failure for physicians to continue considering reasonable alternatives to a diagnosis once an initial diagnosis was made.

Graber (2007) described three common pitfalls with defective synthesis of available information:

Context errors when the physician erroneously limits his consideration to only one set of diagnostic possibilities. Example: A patient complains of epigastric pain and the physician fails to consider a heart attack.

Availability errors occur where the physician goes for the most likely or familiar choice over conditions that are less likely or rare. Example: The patient is diagnosed with a migraine when he actually has a brain tumor.

Premature closure means that once the physician has identified a reasonable condition, she does not consider other possibilities. Example: The patient has a gastrointestinal upset; the physician makes the diagnoses of gastroenteritis and the patient experiences a ruptured appendix.

AHRQ reported two promising approaches to reduce cognitive errors. The first involved the process of perfecting performance feedback; the second involved improving physician skills in the ability to monitor and to understand their own thought processes.

Nurses' Decision Making and Medical Errors

There is a paucity of research studies on the types of errors that nurses make in the clinical setting related to cognitive reasoning.

Benner's *Novice to Expert model* (1984) described competency as a continuum from novice to expert. The novice nurse is the inexperienced nurse. An example of this pertains to the new graduate of nursing who has no experience in the workplace and has to learn psychomotor tasks and problem-solve situations in which he or she has no experience to draw from.

The expert nurse has performed the psychomotor tasks numerous times and does not have to think about them when they are done; also, she or he has experience to draw from when taking care of patients. He or she intuitively knows the right action based on previous experience and application of knowledge in the present situation.

Tucker and Edmondson (2002) from Harvard Business School identified two types of process failures: problems and errors. They defined error as "the execution of a task that is either unnecessary or incorrectly carried out and that could have been avoided with appropriate distribution of preexisting information." They defined a problem as "a disruption in a worker's ability to execute a prescribed task because the worker does not have something he/she needs at that time to perform the task or something is present that should not be and interferes with the designated task." Nurses experience problems and errors constantly.

The researchers obtained qualitative data resulting from 239 hours of observation of 26 nurses at nine hospitals followed by interviews for 12 nurses at seven of the hospitals in the sample. They reported that there were 194 failures during their observations. Problems made up the largest portion (166) of these data; 88 percent of the problems surfaced as the nurses were preparing to care for the patient; 91 percent of the problems resulted from a breakdown in information or material transfer to the nurse. In five of the interviews conducted, the nurses stated that many problems they experience arise from other groups or departments. Examples included dealing with central supply and housekeeping.

There were 28 errors observed that fell into three categories:

Incorrect actions made by the nurse (39 percent). Example: The nurse forgot to administer medications to a patient for the entire shift.

Errors made by other staff (18 percent). Example: Nurses having to correct an incorrect diet entry from a previous shift.

Unnecessary actions resulting from faulty processes flows (43 percent). Example: Nurses preparing a patient for transfer to discover a reversal of the decisions.

Tucker and Edmondson emphasized the importance of distinguishing problems from errors; problems were visible and frequent, which makes them amenable for improvement without being interpersonally threatening. Errors were described as first-order problem solving. First-order problem solving actions resolve the immediate problem, as in getting the needed supplies for the patient, but do not address the underlying causes for the problem to prevent reoccurrence. First-order problem solving can be counterproductive because the problems might not be reported and then the underlying causes are not improved. Also, first-order problem solving can create problems in another area. The example given was when the nurse borrows linens or other supplies from another ward, then that ward experiences linen shortages. This study reported that 33 minutes on average per 8-hour shift were wasted by nurses trying to cope with system failures.

Nurses were reported to problem solve with their peers, people who were socially close; notification of physicians or managers were rare. Nurses requested assistance from managers or physicians only 7 percent of the time.

Second-order problem solving involves taking action to address underlying causes. Even when any behavior that called attention to the situation was classified as second-order problem solving, only 7 percent of the nurses met this criteria. One nurse was reported as saying "I do not feel my voice is heard."

The researchers argued that the nurses' decision making and failure to report problems for handling the underlying issues were most likely due to the emphasis on individual accountability in health care, efficiency demands at the unit level, and empowerment or widely shared goal of developing units that can function without any direct managerial assistance.

They concluded by stating that both errors and problems can be detected and used as starting points for organizational learning and improvement and that managers have an essential role in assisting with problem-solving efforts and providing worker support.

In time, problems and errors would be viewed as sources of learning and workers would be valued by managers as proactive and motivated employees.

Tucker and Spear (2006) sampled a cross-sectional group of six U.S. hospitals and looked at the frequency of work system failures and their impact on nurse productivity. Work system failures are called operational failures defined by the "inability of the work system to reliably provide information services, and supplies when, where, and to whom needed." They reported an average of 8.4 work system failures per every 8-hour shift. The top five most frequent work system failures involved medications, supplies, orders, staffing, and equipment. For an average 8-hour shift, nurses spent an average task time of only 3.1 minutes; however, nurses were interrupted mid-task an average of eight times per shift. Tucker and Spear recommended that designing robust processes where nurses are not interrupted could help prevent errors.

Recently, Westbrook, Woods, Rob, Dunsmuir, and Day (2010) compared observational data with patient's medication charts using a volunteer sample of 98 nurses from six wards in two major teaching hospitals who were observed administering 4,271 medications to 720 patients over 505 hours. The study divided the results into two categories of errors. Procedural failures involved issues such as a break in aseptic technique. Clinical errors involved issues such as the wrong dose of a medication administered.

Each interruption was associated with a 12.1 percent increase in procedural failures and a 12.7 percent increase in clinical errors. Interruptions occurred in 53.1 percent of medication administrations, and the estimated risk of a major error was estimated at 2.3 percent; when there were four interruptions, this risk doubled to 4.7 percent. The authors concluded that among these nurses at these two hospitals, the occurrence and frequency of interruptions were significantly associated with the incidence of procedural failures and clinical errors.

A sentinel article by Murphy, Emmett, Ruch, Pepicello, and Murphy (1997) studied more than 170,000 health care workers including 47,692 registered nurses in 138 acute care settings. They reported that the role of the registered nurses was characterized by numerous excessive tasks, a loss of focus on nursing components, and a significant overlap of roles with other job categories.

The characteristics reported were related to decreased morale and decreased physician–patient satisfaction with care, and resulted in increased health care costs. The authors suggested a need for leaders to "develop new methods for controlling the complexity of healthcare systems; specifically, the registered nurse role."

Nurses working on the front line work with fewer staff, and as a result, their decision making is confined to getting the shift work done to meet the needs of the patient during a compressed time period. Because of the increased complexity at the unit level, nurses are often isolated and rushed when problem solving to meet the most urgent goals.

Nurses make mistakes in assigning nursing diagnoses to patients according to studies from 1966 to 2006, which described wide variation in nurses' interpretations of clinical data (Lunney, 2008). Because inaccurate data interpretation or misdiagnoses can lead to unexpected and undesirable outcomes, Lunney advocated addressing the issue of accuracy in nurses' diagnosis.

Decision making at all levels of the system affect patient safety. To make better decisions, transparency is needed. To have transparency, a patient safety culture is needed.

Crew Resource Management Training

Crew Resource Management Training was traced back to a workshop, Resource Management on the Flight Deck, which was held by the National Aeronautics and Space Administration (NASA) in 1979, according to Helmreich, Merritt, and Wilhelm (1999). At this workshop, the label of Cockpit Resource Management (CRM) was made for the process of training crews in a manner that would reduce pilot error by making better use of human resources on the flight deck. Research presented at this conference identified the human-error aspects for the majority of air crashes: failures of interpersonal communications, decision making, and leadership. Since that time, CRM training programs have grown in the United States and globally.

AHRQ (n.d.-c) recognized that for many years the aviation industry had required crew members to receive specific training in how to work as a team. Several studies have documented the poor levels of teamwork in medicine. Areas such as the operating room had a culture where surgeons were significantly less likely to acknowledge their own fatigue level or accept any suggestions from junior staff. This was seen as similar to pilots.

Teamwork training focuses on effective communication skills to create a more collaborative and cohesive work environment and, most importantly, create a work climate in which all staff feel comfortable to speak up when they observe what might be a potential risk or problem. Team training involves establishing processes to cross-check each team member's actions, offer assistance when needed, and address errors in a neutral fashion that is not construed as judgmental.

Team training emphasizes the role of human factors: effects of fatigue, perceptual errors, and the impact of various management styles and organizational cultures.

As mentioned in previous chapters, the most-often-cited team training program in health care is the Team STEPPS, a collaborative effort by the U.S. Department of Defense and the AHRQ.

Team STEPPS was based on more than 20 years of research and lessons from the application of teamwork principles. It involves a curriculum, a toolkit, and an easy-to-use multimedia kit that contains the fundamental modules, pocket guide, video vignettes that illustrate key concepts, and workshop materials that include a supporting CD and DVD.

The program has three phases based on lessons learned, the literature of quality and patient safety, and culture change. The first phase is for assessment of the organization's readiness for starting the Team

STEPPS training and involves need analysis; the second phase relates to planning, training, and implementation; and the third phase is to sustain and spread improvements in teamwork, performance, clinical processes, and outcomes that result from the Team STEPPS initiative.

There is an abundance of tested team training tools that can be ordered for free at this Web site, including the Team STEPPs Rapid Response Systems (RRS) Training module and questionnaires for how individuals measure the current state of teamwork within their organization. Available at: http://teamstepps.ahrq.gov/abouttoolsmaterials.htm

Currently, the Joint Commission's Universal Protocol involves a mandatory "time-out" where all team members participate in the review of the details of the surgery that is about to take place. Health care organizations are also coupling teamwork requirements into structuring communication requirements, such as SBAR training.

Studies in teamwork training have produced inconsistent results. The studies have produced consistent results for improvements in the participants' knowledge of teamwork principles, attitudes toward the importance of teamwork, and improvement in the overall safety climate. These results have not yet necessarily translated into sustainable behavioral changes or improved skills (AHRQ, n.d.).

Anesthesia Crisis Resource Management (ACRM) is a simulated realistic enactment that uses scenarios of operating room incidents followed by rapid cycle, learner-centered debriefings using videotapes of the clinical team's performance. It was developed by David Gaba and colleagues at Stanford University in collaboration with the Palo Alto Veteran Affairs Medical Center. It was designed to assist anesthesiologists to work in multidisciplinary teams to better effectively manage crisis events.

The multidisciplinary team included physicians, nurses, technicians, and other medical professionals. The aim was to enable the trainees to learn from adverse clinical occurrences and to be able to work in a more effective manner with various leadership, followership, and communication styles. This curriculum comprises 3 days of simulation training. The simulated operating room includes actual monitoring equipment, a full patient simulator, a video station for recording the team's performance, and a debriefing room.

There are several instructors that run the ACRM scenarios. After the ACRM training, a yearly refresher is done. The ACRM training is currently used at several major teaching institutions in the United States and globally.

MedTeams is another team training program that was designed to decrease medical errors through interdisciplinary teamwork. It was originally created by the Dynamics Research Corporation (DRC) for emergency departments on the premise that most errors occur as the result of breakdowns in the systems-level defenses. Each member is expected to take an assertive role in breaking the error chain. Each core team includes at least a physician and a nurse. DRC identified from needs-analysis work, five critical dimensions with 48 specific and observable behaviors that were linked to effective teamwork.

They constructed Behaviorally Anchored Rating Scales (BARS) for each of the behaviors. They also included expert panel review and modification of the curriculum based on that review. Training consists of an 8-hour training session and a 4-hour practicum session (Baker, Gustafson, Beaubien, Salas, & Barach, 2005).

The critical success factors for organizations thinking about embarking on team training programs were reported by Almeida et al. (2009) as

The team training should be aligned with organizational objectives, safety aims, and organizational goals.

There needs to be organizational support for the team training initiative. This means time, money, and leadership's active involvement.

Frontline care leaders need to be on board and support the training. As informal leaders, they can either be the source for support or the resistance in training efforts.

The environment needs to be prepared along with the trainees for team training.

The resources need to be determined along with time commitment and availability.

There needs to be facilitation for application of trained teamwork skills on the job.

The effectiveness measures need to be developed and measurement needs to be done for evaluation of the program with feedback to the leadership and staff.

So why are team training and better communication difficult processes to implement in health care systems?

Lee (2010) stated that working in teams does not come easily to physicians. Physicians still see themselves as the heroic lone healers. Physicians now need to be both team leaders and team players. This is a huge shift in roles, where not that long ago nurses were not regarded as professionals but as technicians whose jobs mainly comprised following physician orders.

Lee provided the success story of Geisinger Health care system, where hospital re-admissions were cut by 50 percent. Geisinger utilized nurses as care coordinators and placed them in the offices of patients' primary care physicians. These nurses continually assess this group of patients to identify the patients that can be handled by them and those who need to be seen by the physicians instead. This entails giving nurses quite a lot of responsibility for managing this group of patients. The results speak for themselves: a 50 percent reduction in re-admissions.

Lee argued that the teamwork required in organizations will depend on the leadership's ability to either inspire or require teamwork. He stated that teamwork provides a competitive advantage and is difficult to implement due to the physician's culture of autonomy. He stated that cultural barriers for physicians relate to their resistance to being measured, their need to be perfect, and their reluctance to criticize their colleagues. Physician autonomy, which is cherished by physicians, is not synonymous with quality.

CONCLUSION

As microsystems are designed at the unit level, consideration of the cultural components, team performance, and how well the various groups respectfully interact with each other is essential for successful patient safety efforts. There is wide variation in the cultures within a health care organization.

Both nurses and physicians make errors in decision making. There needs to be more emphasis in this area for research. Nurses' roles are complex and interdependent, with significant overlap of roles and tasks with other health care professionals. Nurses also solve a lot of problems at the unit level and do not report these events for system improvement.

Physicians make diagnostic errors and many of these errors go undetected. Programs that provide feedback in the ability to monitor and to understand their own thought processes may be useful as a means to reduce these types of errors.

Nurses must be fully supported by administration and physician leaders to implement patient-centered care. Staff that are fearful to speak up when they see a concern, become a risk point for the patient. Staff who put their egos ahead of the needs of the patient should not be tolerated. Unfortunately, due to hierarchies, power gradients, and personalities, these types of unacceptable behaviors have been tolerated and accepted with silence.

Team training has proliferated, particularly for areas of high risk and fast pace such as operating rooms, emergency rooms, and labor and delivery areas. Team training assists staff with developing a better safety climate. All of the programs need to have measurements for effectiveness of the training. There are three primary models for disclosure. To have an engaged workforce means that staff must have trust that they can speak up to do the right thing for patients. Disruptive and disrespectful behaviors that are accepted are not conducive to developing a patient safety culture.

REFERENCES

Agency for Healthcare Research and Quality. (2009). *Hospital survey on patient safety culture: 2009 comparative database report.* Retrieved July 4, 2010, from http://www.ahrq.gov/qual/hospsurvey09/

Agency for Healthcare Research and Quality. (n.d.-a). *Perspectives on safety: In conversations with.. J. Bryan Sexton PhD, MA.* Retrieved February 20, 2011, from http://www.webmm.ahrq.gov/perspective.aspx?perspectiveID=34

Agency for Healthcare Research and Quality. (n.d.-b). *Patient safety primer: Safety culture.* Retrieved February 11, 2011, from http://psnet.ahrq.gov/primer.aspx?primerID=5

Agency for Healthcare Research and Quality. (n.d.-c). *Patient safety primer: Teamwork training.* Retrieved July 30, 2010, from http://psnet.ahrq.gov/primer.aspx?primerID=8

American Nurses Association. (2001). *ANA Code of Ethics for Nurses.* Retrieved February 10, 2011, from http://docs.google.com/viewer?a=v&q=cache:MMbvQG3ZkykJ:www.bioethicscourse.info/codesite/ANA%2520Code%2520of%2520Ethics%2520for%2520Nurses.doc+ana+code+of+ethics&hl=en&gl=us&pid=bl&srcid=ADGEESiEPwoDa27KKMMxALIbStVe5VwxLUVgkaR7MdBN2Z4lKb-_m4TqrqcIbhfMIeVTjhAOEd-M_Xi3bfZ9rMF4aTcuQzkqcDx2NnssTbaTBwCS8aiVzZyIURW1mCGhMKzax89qchmk&sig=AHIEtbQleedZrj03IlgrnxYlnoRqBJm8zg

American Nurses Credentialing Center. *Find a Magnet facility.* Retrieved February 20, 2011, from http://www.nursecredentialing.org/Magnet/FindaMagnetFacility.aspx

American Society for Healthcare Risk Management. (2003). *Disclosure of unanticipated events; the next step in better communication with patients. First of three parts.* ASHRM monograph. Retrieved June 5, 2010, from http://

www.premierinc.com/quality/tools-services/safety/topics/patient_safety/sample-policies.jsp

American Society for Healthcare Risk Management. (2003). *Disclosure of unanticipated events: Creating an effective patient communication policy. Second of three parts.* ASHRM monograph. Retrieved June 5, 2010, from http://www.premierinc.com/quality/tools-services/safety/topics/patient_safety/sample-policies.jsp

American Society for Healthcare Risk Management. (2004) *Disclosure: What works now & What can work even better. Third of three parts.* ASHRM monograph. Retrieved June 5, 2010, from http://www.premierinc.com/quality/tools-services/safety/topics/patient_safety/sample-policies.jsp

Baker, D. P., Gustafson, S., Beaubien, J. M., Salas, E., & Barach, P. (2005). *Medical team training programs in healthcare.* Retrieved August 1, 2010, from http://www.ncbi.nlm.nih.gov/bookshelf/br.fcgi?book=aps4&part=A7246

Baum, K. (n.d.). *Commentary: Why evidence-based medicine is a key component of patient safety.* United Health Foundation. Retrieved June 1, 2010, from http://www.unitedhealthfoundation.org/download/

Beach, M., Saha, S., & Cooper, L. A. (2006). The role and relationship of cultural competence and patient-centeredness in health care quality. *Commonwealth Fund.* Retrieved June 5, 2010, from http://www.commonwealthfund.org/Search.aspx?search=patient+centeredness

Benner, P. (1984). *From novice to expert: Excellence and power in clinical practice.* Menlo Park, CA: Addison Wesley.

Berwick, D. (2009). *What 'patient-centered' should mean: Confessions of an extremist.* Retrieved July 8, 2010, from http://content.healthaffairs.org/cgi/content/abstract/28/4/w555

CBC News. (2009, November, 7). *Admitting errors reduces them: Montreal hospital Province to use Jewish General as model for creating registry of incidents.* Retrieved June 5, 2010, from http://www.cbc.ca/canada/montreal/story/2009/11/06/jgh-mistakes-registry.html

Cooper, J. R. M., Walker, J. T., Winters, K., Williams, R., Askew, R., & Robinson, J. C. (2009). Nursing students' perceptions of bullying behaviors by classmates. *Issues in Educational Research, 19*(3), pp. 212–226.

Committee on Quality of Health care in America, Institute of Medicine. (2001). *Crossing the quality chasm: A new health system for the 21st century.* Washington, DC: National Academy Press.

Desautels, C. (n.d.). *Consultation &services for members and non-planetree members.* Retrieved July 4, 2010, from http://www.planetree.org/consultation.html

Dickey, J., Daminao, R. J., & Ungerleider, R. (2003). Our surgical culture of blame: A time for change. *Journal of Thoracic and Cardiovascular Surgery, 126*, pp. 1259–1260.

Fein, S., Hillborne, L., Kagawa-singer, M., Spiritus, E., Keenan, C., Seymann, G., ... Wenger, N. A. (2005). A conceptual model for disclosure of medical errors. In: Advances in patient safety: From research to implementation (Volume 2, pp. 483-94). Rockville, MD: Agency for Healthcare Research and Quality. (AHRQ Publication No. 05-0021-2).

Fleming, M. (2005). Patient safety culture measurement and improvement: A "how to" guide. *Healthcare Quarterly, 8*, pp. 14–19.

Foster, T. C., Johnson, J. K., Nelson, E. C., & Batalden, P. B. (2007). *Using a Malcolm Baldridge framework to understand high performing clinical microsystems.* Retrieved January, 2, 2011, from http://docs.google.com/viewer?a=v&q=cache:R7WReXc8fCEJ:clinicalmicrosystem.org/toolkits/getting_started/baldrige_microsystems.pdf+baldridge+model+and+microsystems&hl=en&gl=us&pid=bl&srcid=ADGEESjQU406LubYgT8dreGkMiJZ_QzBAh5npKKvt7tpgPsz_DIJmp01zwRjxQuC74rQ3K0Fbn4FWOyfifTbvXe9mrxBnC3WxwNDz81AFcm-ozcQZ6QNHTSVwZ4zOYmgXQ08KcbbSjaW&sig=AHIEtbSV8GKl2URypZ5PgaplEUbfDOY0tw

Frampton, S. (2009). Patients first: Creating a patient-centered system. *American Journal of Nursing, 109*(3), pp. 30–33.

Gallagher, T. H., Garbutt, J. M., Waterman, A. D., Flum, D. R., Larson, E. B., Waterman, B. M., ... Levinson, W. (2006). Choosing your words carefully: How physicians would disclose harmful medical errors to patients. *Archive Internal Medicine, 166*(15), pp. 1585–1593.

Graber, M. L. (n.d.). AHRQ: *Perspectives on safety: Diagnostic errors in medicine: What do doctors and umpires have in common?* Retrieved June 1, 2010, from http://www.webmm.ahrq.gov/perspective.aspx?perspectiveID=36

Graber, M. L., Franklin, N., & Gordon, F. N. (2005). Diagnostic error in Internal medicine. *Archives of Internal Medicine, 165*(13), pp. 1493–1499.

Groopman, J. (2007). *How physicians think.* New York: Houghton Mifflin Co.

Halverson, D. (2010, February 20). *Abuse in the medical workplace: Fact vs. myth.* Utah Nurse. Retrieved June 5, 2010, from http://www.workplacebullying.org/2010/02/20/medical-workplace/

Helmreich, R. I., Merritt, A. C., & Wilhelm, J. A. (1999) The evolution of Crew Resource Management training in commercial aviation. *International Journal of Aviation Psychology, 9*(1), pp. 19–32.

Institute for Healthcare Improvement. (n.d.). *Clinical microsystem assessment tool.* Retrieved February 11, 2011, from http://www.ihi.org/IHI/Topics/Improvement/ImprovementMethods/Tools/ClinicalMicrosystemAssessmentTool.htm

Isaac, T., Zaslavsky, A.M., Cleary, P.D., & Landon. B.E., (2010). The relationship between patients' perception of care and measures of hospital quality and safety. *Health Services Research.* Aug, *45*(4). 1024–1040.

Joint Commission. (2008). *Sentinel event alert: Behaviors that undermine a culture of safety.* Retrieved June 5, 2010, from http://www.jointcommission.org/sentinelevents/sentineleventalert/sea_40.htm

Kalish, B. J., & Begeny, S. (2007). *Structural barriers to change and innovation in nursing.* Retrieved August 1, 2010, from http://garysalton.blogspot.com/2007/04/structural-barriers-to-change-and.html

Kohn,L.T., Corrigan. J.M., & Donaldson, M.S. (Eds) (2000). *To err is human: Building a safer healthcare system.* Washington DC: National Academy Press

Lachman, V. D. (2006). *Applied ethics in nursing.* New York: Springer.

Lam, R. M., Studdert, D. M., Bohmer, R. M., Berwick, D. M., & Brennan, T. A. (2003). Hospital disclosure practices; results of a national survey: Most hospitals disclose harm to patients at least some of the time, this 2002 survey finds. *Health Affairs, 22*(2), pp. 73–83.

Lee, T. (2010). *Turning doctors into leaders—a message for all of us.* The Center for Global Leadership. Retrieved August 1, 2010, from http://centerforgloballeadership.wordpress.com/2010/04/09/turning-doctors-into-leaders-a-message-for-all-of-us/

Lundmark, V. A. (2008). *Chapter 46: Magnet environments for professional nursing practice.* Retrieved July 4, 2010, from http://search.ahrq.gov/search?q=lundmark+magnet&entqr=0&output=xml_no_dtd&proxystylesheet=AHRQ_GOV&client=AHRQ_GOV&site=default_collection

Lunney, M. (2008). Critical need to address accuracy of nurses' diagnoses. *OJIN.* Retrieved June 1, 2010, from http://www.nursingworld.org/MainMenuCategories/ANAMarketplace/ANAPeriodicals/OJIN/TableofContents/vol132008/No1Jan08/ArticlePreviousTopic/AccuracyofNursesDiagnoses.aspx

Mohr, J. J., Batalden, P., & Barach, P. (2004). Integrating patient safety into the clinical microsystems. *Quality Safe Health Care.* Retrieved January, 20, 2011, from http://www.ncbi.nlm.nih.gov/pmc/articles/PMC1765806/pdf/v013p0ii34.pdf

Murphy, B. E., Emmett, C., Ruch, S., Pepicello, J., & Murphy, M. (1997). *Managing an increasingly complex system.* Nursing Management. Retrieved June 1, 2010, from http://journals.lww.com/nursingmanagement/Abstract/1997/10010/Managing_an_Increasingly_Complex_System.9.aspx

O'Brien, S. J. (2000, October 16). *The Bully Boss.* Retrieved February 1, 2011, from http://www.workplacebullying.org/press/waco1.html

Planetree. (2010, July 19). *Planetree receives Commonwealth fund grant to develop designation criteria and measurement strategies for person-centered care.* Retrieved August 1, 2010, from http://planetree.org/News.html

Robert Wood Johnson Foundation. (2003). *What Front-line caregivers need to succeed.* Retrieved Feb 20, 2011, from http://www.rwjf.org/reports/grr/036103.htm

Rowell, P. A. (2010). *Lateral violence: Nurse against nurse.* ANA. Retrieved June 5, 2010, from http://www.nursingworld.org/mods/mod440/lateral full.htm#role

Salas, E., Almeida, S. A., Salisbury, M., King, H., Lazzara, E. H., Lyons, R., ... McQuillan, R. (2009) What are the critical success factors for team training in health care? *Journal Quality Patient Safety,* 35(8), pp. 398–405.

Senge, P. (1999). *The dance of change: The challenges of sustaining momentum in learning.* New York: Double Day.

Sexton, J. B., Helmreich, R. L., Neilands, T. B., Rowan, K., Vella, K., Boyden, J., ... Thomas, E. J. (2006).*The safety attitudes questionnaire: Psychometric properties, benchmarking data, and emerging research.* Retrieved 1 June, 2010, from http://www.psnet.ahrq.gov/resource.aspx?resourceID=3601

Tucker, A. L., & Edmondson, A. C. (2002). *Why hospitals don't learn from failures: Organizational and psychological dynamics that inhibit system change.* Harvard Business School. Retrieved June 1, 2010, from http://docs.google.com/viewer?a=v&q=cache:iisoXOSBZ1QJ:www.npsf.org/standup/members/download/articles-whyhospitals.pdf+Tucker,+A.+L.+%26+Edmondson,+A.+C.+(2002).+Why+hospitals+don't+learn+from+failures:+Organizati onal+and+psychological+dynamics+that+inhibit+system+change.&hl=en &gl=us&pid=bl&srcid=ADGEEShpah-uDr34srT3yVNt4huuwuDw4cZ dhSLG6SYTZcOI5TygXP1baieD5g3inrk8eutLNS-OGCiO1Xfea1-uyjkKJq egSW6UG5jlUhq0qNxBgWNR6ndqiDeg5bwvsCIkY180fPvp&sig=AHIE tbRsIYT6bt9Lo5SrjPyGmdzECJyJMg

Tucker, A. L., & Spear, S. J. (2006). Operational failures and interruptions in hospital nursing. *Health Services Research.* Retrieved October 20, 2011, from http://www.ncbi.nlm.nih.gov/pmc/articles/PMC1713207/

Westbrook, J. I., Woods, A., Rob, M. I., Dunsmuir, W. T., & Day, R. O. (2010). Association of interruptions with an increased risk and severity of medication administration errors. *Archives of Internal Medicine, 170*(8), pp. 683–690.

Wilbert, B., & Itoigawa, N. (Eds.). (2001). *Safety culture in nuclear power operations.* New York: Taylor & Francis.

Witman, A. B., Park, D. M., & Hardin, S. B. (1996). How do patients want physicians to handle mistakes? A survey on internal medicine patients in an academic setting. *Archives of Internal Medicine, 156*(22), pp. 2565–2569.

Workplace Bullying Institute (WBI). (2010). *Results of the 2010 WBI U.S. workplace bullying survey.* Retrieved February 2, 2011, from http://www.workplacebullying.org/research/WBI-NatlSurvey2010.html

11

Design at the Individual Level

The IOM's report *Crossing the Quality Chasm: A New Health System for the 21st Century* stated that health care has six aims: safety, effectiveness, timeliness, efficiency, equitability, and patient centeredness (see Figure 11.1). As these outcome dimensions can be measured, the system should be aligned to achieve them. For this to occur, the system design at the individual level should mirror the desired outcomes. In effect, the entire care environment should be designed according to IOM's six aims. To enable the employee to be more patient centered, the leadership designs the work environment to be employee centered, so that the employee is fully engaged in his or her work. This means that the work environment should be designed in a manner that strives to enhance the QWL.

All staff members bring their views of the world, ethics, values, beliefs, and competencies to the organization. Competencies are the knowledge, skills, and attitudes needed to perform a role. The leadership shapes and designs the environment for patient safety at the individual level just as they do at the microsystem level. This means that the environment needs to be shaped in a manner that provides every opportunity for staff to succeed and not fail. A review of each of these elements is presented.

FIGURE 11.1
System design of the IOM six aims at the individual level.

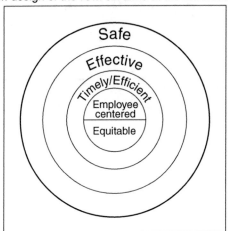

SAFE

Safety is the basic level that staff should expect when they work in health care. Unsafe work conditions place staff at risk for personal and/or psychological injury.

Leaders must design the work environment to be safe for individuals. No employee should suffer a preventable injury, workplace violence, or psychological threats. Cost containment measures have left nurses feeling abandoned, burned out, and frustrated at having to do so much more with so much less.

How is the work environment critical to patient safety? Nurses are on the front line all of the time, 7 days a week. Admissions occur 24/7. Patients are being admitted sicker and they are discharged quicker, so the next patient can be admitted. Nursing work processes such as medication administration are often designed in a manner that is conducive to errors. Medication rooms are frequently areas of high traffic, noise, and numerous distractions and each of these characteristics may lead to nursing errors.

I have worked in a hospital with chronic staffing shortage, and where housekeeping was subcontracted. Needle-stick injuries occurred because housekeeping did not empty the needle containers in a timely fashion. When the nurse would go to discard a needle, she or he would find the container full.

Nurses encounter numerous distractions and interruptions. Medication administration requires the nurse's full attention to prevent medication errors. Potter et al. (2005) conducted a study funded from a grant by the AHRQ on HFE techniques combined with qualitative observations to analyze the working conditions that contribute to medical errors in the acute care setting. Human Factor Engineering (HFE) assists in reducing medical errors, including cognitive errors related to poor person–machine interfaces.

Researchers have developed cognitive pathways, which are visual graphics that demonstrate the patterns of nurses' work and the relationships that interruptions and cognitive overload may have on omissions and errors in providing care. Each activity carried out by the nurse has been coded into one of five steps of the nursing process: assessment, diagnosis, planning, intervention, and evaluation.

There were seven registered nurses observed for 43 hours by the researchers. The activities and time each nurse took was observed and categorized. The breakdown was as follows: consultation was the highest (26 percent), followed by patient contact (25 percent), documentation (23 percent), and medication preparation and administration (16 percent). Searching for supplies and other items was observed at 5 percent. The cognitive pathways drawn demonstrated that the nurses' work was nonlinear in nature and complex.

Based on the cognitive pathway analysis, interruptions occurred 7 percent of the nurses' work time. Nurses were frequently interrupted during interventional work such as nursing assessments, administering medications, problem-solving IV medications, and patient teaching. Of particular note in the study was the design of the medication room. In most cases, medication rooms are highly visible and contain high levels of traffic. This study emphasized the need for further research into the nature of nurses' cognitive work and better design systems to reduce errors or omissions.

The AHRQ sponsored a research project published in May 2003 that has led to many further research studies and questions regarding work environment conditions on the effects of patient safety. Hickman et al. (2003) summarized evidence on the effects of health care working conditions on patient safety. Working conditions were categorized into five areas:

1. Workforce staffing
2. Work-flow design
3. Personal/social factors

4. Physical environment

5. Organizational factors

    Workforce staffing refers to the expected job assignments of the health care workers. It comprises four key aspects: volume of the work assigned, professional skills required for the job assigned, duration of experience for the job assigned, and effects of work schedules assigned.

    Work flow design focuses on the processes that must occur to deliver health care to patients. This involves the interactions between the workers and the interactions with the workers and the workplace environment.

    Personal/social focuses on the personal, social, and professional aspects of the health care work environment. Personal factors relate to stress, motivation, burnout, dissatisfaction, and control over the work assigned. Social factors relate to interrelationships among workers such as role ambiguity, group status, conflict, and support behaviors.

    Physical environment working conditions focuses on the physical features of the environment that either enhance the work flow to be done safely or may create unsafe conditions for the work to be done. This includes lighting, noise levels, physical layout, and any other physical characteristics that support the work.

    Organizational factors have both formal and informal characteristics. These refer to type of health care institution (teaching, community, and private), culture, level of centralization and decentralization, and so on.

    The researchers conducted extensive literature reviews from five major databases resulting in a total of 23,179 citations. They ranked the quality of evidence using the U.S. Preventive Services Task Force, *The Guide to Community Preventive Services*, the Oxford Centre for Evidence-Based Medicine, and AHRQ Evidence Report/Technology Assessment Number 47, *Systems to Rate the Strength of Scientific Evidence*. The research studies were graded on design suitability and assessment of strength of evidence using a three-tier approach.

AHRQ Results on Nurse Staffing

Events that were nonfatal such as decubitus ulcers and patient falls had a plausible direct relationship to the numbers of nursing staff in both acute care and nursing home settings. Lower nurse–patient staffing ratios were associated with higher rates of nonfatal events. Mortality due to nurse staffing was reported as an imperfect measure due to the confounding issue of dealing with preventable or nonpreventable causes.

There was sufficient evidence to conclude that higher nursing workload is associated with higher incidence of medication errors and that the effect of nursing workload on outcomes differs between intensive care and nonintensive care settings.

AHRQ Results on Physician Workload

The majority of studies were limited to physicians performing technical procedures such as surgery and cardiology. There was sufficient evidence that higher physician workload was associated with lower hospital mortality rates, but there was not enough evidence to support whether physician workload affected the rate of medical errors. Nor was there sufficient evidence to prove that physician workload affected the rate of recognition of medical errors after they occurred. There was also insufficient evidence to conclude that complexity influences the rate of adverse events.

AHRQ Results on Professional Qualifications (Physician)

There was sufficient evidence to conclude that physicians with specialty training do experience lower rates of fatal and nonfatal adverse outcomes for certain procedures and medical conditions. There was insufficient evidence as to whether physician specialty affected the rate of medical errors or the rate of recognition of medical errors after they occurred. Also, there was insufficient evidence to determine if the complexity of the care plan affected whether physician specialty affected patient outcomes related to patient safety.

AHRQ Results on Professional Experience (Nurse)

There was insufficient or no evidence to demonstrate that professional experience affected patient outcomes related to patient safety. There was insufficient evidence to determine if professional experience affected the rate of medical errors.

AHRQ Results on Professional Experience (Physician)

Three studies were examined and none demonstrated that more experience in performing surgical procedures was associated with lower rates of postoperative complications. The studies suggested that the participation of training students in surgical procedures that were supervised by senior surgeons was not associated with higher complication rates; however, this was too low a number from which to draw conclusions.

AHRQ Results on Scheduling (Temporal Factors) Physicians and Nurses

The researchers acknowledged that work schedules and work shifts have received attention and much of the attention has come from other research conducted in fields such as aviation. Physician resident training schedules have been a focus for study of fatigue; however, the literature review concluded that there was limited evidence that fatigue caused higher rates of errors when repetitive tasks and tasks requiring extended vigilance were performed.

There was insufficient or no evidence to conclude that temporal factors affect patient outcomes that are related to patient safety, affect the rate of medical errors, or the rate of recognition of medical errors after they occur.

AHRQ Results on Environmental Factors

The researchers did not identify any supporting association between shared work spaces and medical errors or patient safety. Task complexity was also not covered in this report.

There were no identified studies that supported an association between monotony or redundancy and medical errors or patient safety.

AHRQ Results on Transitions of Care (Handoffs)

There was sufficient evidence to conclude that hospital discharge process employing a dedicated staff and having an outpatient component reduces re-admission rates and hospital days. The evidence was not sufficient to conclude that these programs reduce medical errors and associated adverse events. One study of interest on dispensing medication, from a random sample of over 50,000 Medicare registrants in Quebec in 1990, concluded that the greater the number of prescribing physicians, the greater the risk that the patient received a potentially inappropriate medication.

AHRQ Results on Work-flow Design

The researchers did not find sufficient evidence to conclude that work-flow design factors affected the incidence of adverse outcomes. The researchers concluded there was sufficient evidence that interruptions and distractions are associated with medication dispensing errors; but there was insufficient evidence to demonstrate an association with distractions and interruptions with errors in other areas.

AHRQ RESULTS ON PERSONAL/SOCIAL WORKING CONDITIONS

Organizational stress and job stress were associated with higher malpractice risk and patient falls; however, malpractice events are not a good measure for patient safety, so there was insufficient evidence to conclude that stress caused increases in adverse patient outcomes.

Also, there was insufficient evidence to conclude that stress affected the rate of medical errors. There was no evidence to support that stress affected the rate of recognition after they occur. Burnout and dissatisfaction also had insufficient evidence to support the association with patient outcomes related to patient safety and to prove that they affected the rate of medical errors.

AHRQ Results on Physical Environment

There was insufficient evidence to conclude that noise levels affected patient outcomes that are related to patient safety. The researchers found sufficient evidence from studies to conclude that ambient noise levels did not affect the rate of medication errors.

AHRQ Results on Organizational Working Conditions

There were inconsistent results reported and insufficient evidence to conclude that organizational working conditions affected patient outcomes related to patient safety. The researchers stated that the studies provided a framework for further research in this field. There was insufficient evidence that organizational working conditions affected the rate of medical errors. There was evidence that suggested elements of organizational culture affected error-reporting rates, but there were not enough studies sufficient to answer the question.

Most of the evidence presented was inconclusive, with insufficient support from the research studies to conclude any association with work environment factors and adverse patient outcomes. This is not surprising because patient safety is in its infancy and research studies need to be designed in a manner that seeks the answers to specific patient safety questions. The need for further research and measurements of patient safety variables was emphasized.

Communication to Enhance Patient Safety

The work environment is complex, and effective communication skills are required for all interactions with team members to establish and maintain an effective patient safety culture.

Education of staff at the front line must include communication skills, expected behaviors when interacting with each other, and consequences when the staff member is not compliant. Some units have a code of conduct where all staff who work on the unit draft it, sign it, and hold each other accountable to it. No one is exempt, and feedback on behaviors is expected.

Units may elect to have 360-degree evaluations for nurses and physicians so that they receive feedback on how their behaviors are perceived by their stakeholders.

Bullying behaviors and disruptive behaviors have no place in a professional, caring work environment. Staff should be encouraged to speak up and have a right to expect a safe working environment.

EFFECTIVE

You buy a car and expect it to get you from point A to point B. You would not be happy if the car looked great but did not do what it was designed to do. When processes are effective, it means that the result is as intended. Health care should be effective. This means that the workers need the right tools to provide the right care to the right patient at the right time on a consistent basis.

We want the care that we provide to patients to be effective. For example, all patients should have effective pain management. We measure pain by quantitative pain scores and intervene when the patient experiences pain.

At the individual level, for their actions to be successful, nurses must possess the right knowledge, skills, and attitudes to successfully perform their role. This also means that nurses on the front line need to know the right thing to do at the right time when caring for patients. EBP was defined by Newhouse, Dearholt, Poe, Pugh, and White (2007) as "a problem-solving approach to clinical decision making within a health-care organization that integrates the best available scientific evidence with the best available experiential (patient and practitioner) evidence. EBP considers internal and external influences on practice and encourages critical thinking in the judicious application of evidence to care for the individual patient, patient population, or system."

EBP demands a continual evaluation of the effectiveness of actions. Did the process work as intended? Was the care safe, effective, timely, efficient, equitable, and patient centered? McKenna and McKenna (1999) emphasized that EBP is not the same as research-based practice. EBP comprises a larger domain of information from which the nurse should apply the process of synthesis to sort through information from diverse sources such as expert opinion, past experience, and the patient's response.

Nurses must utilize EBP and not accept nursing rituals just because they have "always done it this way." The goal is to make the best decisions based on the best current evidence. Questioning rituals is essential to developing a new body of knowledge for nursing practice. For example, patients were traditionally warned not to have anything by mouth after midnight before their surgery. Patients are scheduled for surgery the entire next day so some patients may go without anything by mouth for extended periods of time, leading to potential dehydration and other problems.

Schorr (2001) reported that in 1999, the American Society of Anesthesiology (ASA) revised its guidelines about presurgical fasting based on new findings that showed that extended fasting had no benefits in the reduction of stomach contents or acidity. She reported that the new guidelines advise that patients not eat a heavy meal 8 hours prior to surgery but can have a light meal 6 hours prior to surgery, and clear liquids up to 2 hours before surgery. Yet, there are hospitals that force patients to fast for extended periods of time.

The leaders must give the right resources for individuals to do their work. EBP needs a work environment that is supportive of its use in daily practice. Handheld personal digital assistants (PDAs) can contain information that assists with clinical decision making. Enrichment of the work environment by holding interdisciplinary case conferences, nursing conferences, nursing discussions, and mentors for research also assist the individual to implement EBP in the workplace. The Joanna Briggs Institute is one source that has a wealth of accessible information. The organization has a database of current issues for the nurse to critically assess for application in his or her practice. The Web site is www.joannabriggs

.edu.au/about/eb_nursing.php. Also, Johns Hopkins Welch Library has numerous hotlinks to other universities and tutorials on EBP. The Web site is www.welch.jhu.edu/internet/nursing.html# evidence.

Evidence-Based Medicine

Haynes, Devereaus, and Guyatt (2002) stated that evidence-based medicine (EBM) focuses on determining the best research evidence that is relevant to a clinical problem or decision and then applying that evidence to resolve the issue.

Timmermans and Mauck (2005) defined EBM as "the conscientious, explicit, and judicious use of current best evidence in making decisions about the care of individual patients."

Eddy (2005) reported that one problem in the application of EBM is the estimate that only 15 percent of medical practices were based on the gold standard of randomized clinical trials. Eddy stated that the purpose of EBM and clinical practice guidelines was to provide a stronger scientific foundation for "clinical work, to achieve consistency, efficiency, effectiveness, quality, and safety in medical care." He also reported from a national survey where U.S. pediatricians showed that even though approximately 88 percent of them were familiar with asthma guidelines, only 35 percent of them actually followed the guidelines.

Some Web sites that have further information include the Center for Evidence-Based Medicine at www.cebm.net and the Cochrane Collaboration, which contains systematic reviews of the current research, at www.cochrane.org/cochrane-reviews.

The employees must have team training to be competent to work in teams effectively. Along with this is competency in concepts of patient safety: human factors, reliability, disclosure, just culture, RCA, and FMEA.

TIMELY AND EFFICIENT

The work environment either enhances the work or hinders the work. If nurses have to perform ancillary tasks, it decreases their efficiency for providing direct care to patients. Every health care setting has unique challenges in terms of nursing unit locations, linen and supplies set-ups, medication processes, and transport of specimens to the laboratory.

One focus of achieving a timely and efficient environment is the reduction of waste. Nurses may waste time solving problems to get through a shift. For example, they may borrow linen, supplies, or even medications from another nursing unit just to cover the care assigned for a shift. Lean tools focus on eliminating waste. Anything that does not create a product or value to the customer is waste. Increased uses of Lean solutions enable staff to look at processes, break them down into steps, and then eliminate the waste.

The design of the nurses station is changing; for example, decentralized nurses stations are a change for the better. Decentralization saves nurses' time from traveling back and forth to the centralized nurses station. Nurses are in closer proximity to patients.

According to Berczk (2008), more facilities are using Toyota methods that utilize Lean solution to improve every step of care from inventory to discharge. The use of Lean is now becoming the gold standard for U.S. hospitals. Lean solutions reduce inefficiencies in processes by removing waste and leaving value.

Some nurses are distrustful of management, particularly if they have experienced downsizing. They view efficiency projects as one step away from staff reductions. With nursing as the largest salary expense, they know that is possible because it has happened before.

Another aspect of timeliness relates to information. Health care does not do a great job at getting the right information to the right staff at the right time. Performance measures do not belong in meetings where past information is being analyzed. This information needs to be accessible to frontline staff concurrently. How can staff adjust their performance to better care for patients unless they have timely and reliable data? Also, when staff can get concurrent information, they must be empowered to make changes. The leadership must trust that they will do the right thing and allow them to do it. Frequently, even performance improvement teams can make recommendations only to the leadership instead of being empowered to implement the change without going through "the red tape."

EQUITABLE AND EMPLOYEE CENTERED

Equitable

Staff get angry when they discover that pay scales, benefits, and general treatment of certain groups are favored over other groups. Some hospitals have separate physician dining areas, lounges, and parking areas. It would be logical to have interdisciplinary break rooms, lounges, dining rooms, and equitable parking privileges. The work environment can be enriched. One hospital I worked in gave new employees vouchers for free breakfasts during their first week on the job and they had "tea" with the director of nursing (DON) as part of orientation. The DON had the chance to speak informally with all the new staff.

There can be annual events that allow for observation of other team members' roles for a day so that better understanding regarding each other's role in providing patient care can be achieved.

Staff who work on off-shifts such as evening or nights should not feel left out. The leaders should go to them. Regular meetings need to occur on the night shift and on evenings. Project work also needs to occur. Staff should not be left out of working on projects because of work assignments.

Performance evaluations are always a source of dissatisfaction because most of them are very subjective. Also, in the current cost containment environment, many hospitals are giving minimal or no pay raises.

Who gets punished? Disciplinary actions need to be fair and equitable. This means providing a "just culture" and is more difficult to do than one would think. Who determines if a certain behavior was reckless? What about when the behavior was not reckless but a staff member made more than one mistake in a short time? Managers bring their own set of values to the work setting. Some leaders do not provide consistency in punishment when there are medical errors. They do not punish the staff if no harm was done; however, if harm was done, then they punish the staff regardless of whether it was an honest mistake or reckless behavior.

Staff are turning to unions to provide a safe and equitable working environment. The upward trend in union membership may continue if health care leaders do not listen to what staff are telling them.

Employee Centered

Communication: How does leadership communicate with the front line staff? Does the leadership talk *to* staff or talk *with* staff? The leadership for the future will require a new set of skills and effective communication will be essential. Does the leadership listen?

The concept of Patient Safety WalkRounds was a method to get the leadership engaged and have dialog with staff on the front lines. Equally important was the follow-up by the leadership on any actions taken and the feedback to the front line that actions were implemented. Staff is reluctant to speak up when they know that no one is really listening.

Caring: How does the leadership role model caring? Have you ever worked for someone who made you feel special? Your motivation was not about the money. You would work way beyond the normal expectations just because you did not want to let that person down. Caring is a behavior. Forcing nurses to work mandatory overtime on a regular basis, float to areas in which they are not competent, or change work schedules without regard to staff's personal life does not demonstrate caring. In environments where this occurs, nurses feel that they are treated like numbers and not persons. The consequences of this type of treatment are burnout, increased stress, high turnover rates, and disengagement of the workforce.

Empowerment: What degree of empowerment does the leadership allow for staff to make decisions that change practice at the unit level? When nurses are empowered in the workplace and know that they will be supported, it creates a healthier work environment. The leadership needs to provide front line staff with the tools that make it possible to adapt their work environment as needed to provide care. Nurses have the opportunity to lead and integrate the care provided by the teams as new models of nursing care emerge.

Smith (2010) reported on the Glassdoors annual employee survey. The survey is based on 20 questions that address eight workplace topics: work/life balance, career opportunities, communication, compensation and benefits, fairness and respect, employee morale, recognition and feedback, and senior leadership. Facebook was number one with an overall company rating of 4.6 out of a possible of 5. The CEO Zuckerberg achieved a 96 percent approval rating from his employees. Employees commented on the level of work excitement, high level of trust, lack of red tape, and opportunity to jump into projects that interest them. Facebook provides vacation days, free food and transportation, dry cleaning, day care reimbursement, and $4,000 dollars in cash for new parents.

Southwest Airlines came in second on the list with a 4.4 rating and 95 percent approval for the CEO Gary Kelly. Workers have the freedom to dress casual, be creative, and generally have fun on the job. Also, employees and their spouses, eligible dependent children, and parents fly Southwest Airlines for free.

There are also top hospitals and health care systems that were recognized in *Fortune's 100 Best Companies to Work For* list for 2010. There were 14 hospitals or health care systems that earned the recognition in this voluntary program. The list includes Methodist Hospital system in Texas, Baptist Health South in Florida, Scripps Health in California, Ohio Health in Ohio, Kings Daughters Medical Center in Kentucky, and the Mayo Clinic. The ranking results from in-depth employee surveys regarding job satisfaction, working environment, and management's credibility. Wood (2010) included some interview statements from leaders in some of these health care systems, and common themes emerged. The leaders are engaged; they encourage innovation and creativity, and encourage the creation of a healthy work environment.

Unfortunately, there are still hospitals and health care organizations that are far from qualifying as a best place to work. There are nurses and physicians unhappy with their work environment. Some are leaving and trying other jobs. Some of them are staying in the job and carrying their dissatisfaction into the work environment for everyone, including their patients, to see.

Example 1: A nurse working in the oncology department shares her story. She has been in nursing for 20 years. "Administration does not care. The nurse executive just does what the CEO says to do. We have to take care of more patients and have no time for therapeutic communication with them and their families. It is more like assembly-line work. Get the report, line up the treatments and medications, get the vital signs done and hope, really hope, one of your patients doesn't go sour because then you never catch up getting everything done for the rest of the patients you were assigned."

Example 2: A nurse working in the emergency room says that violence has increased there. "We have security guards but the type of patients we come across with mental health issues has risen. Verbal abuse happens more than it should because the patients get frustrated with the waiting times. They don't understand that we have to triage patients and see the sickest first even though we explain it to them on admission to the emergency room. The training residents are difficult. Some of them don't listen to us when we tell them our opinion. My opinion is based on 8 years of emergency room experience. Things happen fast here and it is very frustrating. I think they should increase security here for us but with cost containments, that isn't going to happen."

Example 3: A new graduate laments that she got yelled at when she phoned a physician for orders. "He called me an idiot because I questioned his order. He did this in the hallway by the nurses station so everyone could hear. I struggle to get my work done and frequently end up working into the next shift to get caught up. Some of the other nurses are mean and when I have a question for them, they look at me and ask me why I don't know the answer to that already. I did not learn how to start IVs in nursing school and never got a chance to perform some of the nursing procedures. If the patient has bad veins (and they all seem to have bad veins), I try twice to start the IV, and then have to call another nurse to assist me. I don't know why people have to act like they are so much better than me. I am doing my best and that does not seem to be good enough."

Example 4: A nurse who works on the medical floor has worked there for 5 years. She has resigned and is going to work for home health. "This is a really difficult floor to work. Patients are really sick and the traffic flow from all of the consultants makes it challenging just to keep up with physician orders. Administration does not care about us. We did not get a pay raise last year and this year the maximum is 2 percent. That does not even keep up with the cost of living. At Christmas time, I thought we would get a voucher for a turkey but was told they quit that practice this year. The only positive feedback I get is from my patients. The head nurse doesn't know me. She is in meetings all day. I will be glad to try something new."

Nurses

Employee satisfaction may translate into patient satisfaction, and promotes a healthier work environment. The workplace can be a nurturing environment or a toxic one that can destroy health. According to Faller (2010), one out of every three nurses is dissatisfied with his or her current job. Nearly 30 percent wish to change positions within 1 year, nearly half worry that the job is affecting their health, and only 6 out of 10 would choose nursing as a career if they had it to do over. This was from an AMN Healthcare survey of over 1,400 registered nurses across the country and in various settings. Dissatisfaction translates into a less engaged work force that loses productivity with use of sick time and absenteeism. Also, these individuals are at higher risk for depression.

Physicians

Cedars (2008) reported that a U.S. survey found that 49 percent of 11,950 primary care physicians stated that they want to quit practicing or reduce their patient workload during the next 3 years. The physicians cite frustration with paperwork, complexity of insurance reimbursement, and government regulations.

The costs of employee dissatisfaction can be tremendous. If dissatisfied employees are not working up to their potential, then less work is done on a daily basis and thus increases costs to the organization.

CONCLUSION

To meet the six aims for the health care system, the work environment at the individual level should be safe, effective, timely, efficient, equitable, and employee centered, which facilitates being patient centered. There is much research that needs to be done in the area of patient safety so that learning and better system design occur in a manner that keeps patients and staff safe. The leadership team has an ethical obligation to create and sustain a healthy environment of an engaged work force. This means providing them the right resources, the right working environment, and empowering them to provide safe care for patients, one patient at a time, as part of a working team.

REFERENCES

Berczk, C. (2008, June). The Lean Hospital: More facilities using Toyota methods to improve every step of care from inventory to discharge. *The Hospitalist.* Retrieved February 8, 2011, from http://www.the-hospitalist.org/details/article/186537/The_Lean_Hospital.html

Cedars, D. (2008, November 20). Survey: Half of Primary care physicians dissatisfied: Doctors want to stop practicing or reduce patient load. *7News.* Retrieved February 20, 2011, from http://www.thedenverchannel.com/health/18021241/detail.html

Eddy, D. M. (2005). Evidence-based medicine: A unified approach. *Health Affairs, 24*(1), 9–17.

Faller, M. (2010, February). *Staffing Matters: New survey offers snapshot of nurses' job satisfaction and career plans.* Retrieved February 20, 2011, from http://www.amnhealthcare.com/News/staffing-matters-details.aspx?Id=33432

Haynes, R., Devereaus, P. J., & Guyatt, G. H. (2002). Clinical expertise in the era of evidence-based medicine and patient choice. *Evidence Based Medicine, 7,* 36–38.

Hickman, D. H., Severance, S., Feldstein, A., Ray, L., Garman, P., Schulder. S. S., Hersh, W. R., Krages, K. P., et al. (2003). *The effect of healthcare working conditions on patient safety.* Evidence Report/Technology Assessment

Number 74 (Prepared by Oregon Health & Science University under Contract No 290-97-0018) AHRQ Publication No 03-E031.

McKenna, M. H., & McKenna, P. (1999) Evidence-based practice: Demolishing some myths. *Nursing Standard, 14*(16), pp. 39–42.

Newhouse, R. P., Dearholt, S. L., Poe, S. S., Pugh, L. C., & White, K. M. (2007). *Johns Hopkins nursing evidence-based practice model and guidelines.* Indianapolis, IN: Sigma Theta Tau International.

Potter, P. Wolf, L., Boxerman, S., Grayson, D., Sledge, J., Dunagan, C., Evanoff, B. (2005). Understanding the cognitive work of nursing in the acute care environment. *Journal of Nursing Administration. 35* (7-8). 327–35.

Schorr, M. (2001, May 6). *Patients fasting unnecessarily long before surgery.* Retrieved February 18, 2011 from http://sci.rutgers.edu/forum/show thread.php?t=29615

Smith, J. (2010, December 15). The best companies to work for. *Forbes.* Retrieved January, 10, from http://www.forbes.com/2010/12/14/best-places-to-work-employee-satisfaction-leadership-careers-survey.html

Timmermans, S., & Mauck, A. (2005). The promises and pitfalls of evidence-based medicine. *Health Affairs, 1,* pp. 18–28.

Wood, D. (2010, February). How hospitals achieved their 100 best companies to work for status. *Nursing News.* Retrieved February 1, 2011, from http://www.nursezone.com/nursing-news-events/more-news/How-Hospitals-Achieved-Their-100-Best-Companies-to-Work-For-Status_33390.aspx

IV

*Tools for Building a Better
Reporting System*

12

How the Model Assists Nursing With
Accreditation and Patient Safety Efforts

NURSE EXECUTIVE LEVEL

To date, there has not been an available resource that has current evidence for components of a patient safety and accreditation model for leaders to assess and then decide on a best course of action. The Myers Model for Patient Safety and Accreditation contains the kind and breadth of information that will enable leaders to make decisions to shape the nursing environment of care in a manner that is safe, effective, timely, efficient, equitable, and employee and patient centered.

HOW THE MODEL ASSISTS WITH ACCREDITATION EFFORTS

The Myers Model for Patient Safety and Accreditation presents information on the various accrediting bodies in the United States and internationally. Accreditation allows an objective review of major processes within an organization and identifies opportunities for improvement. The nurse executive can obtain further information and use accreditation as an external driver for selection of improvement projects and maintaining compliance with standards in a manner that increases reliability.

As we have previously noted in this book, accreditation is increasing in the global marketplace as a means to implement quality and patient safety in hospitals.

Within the United States, whole health care networks obtain accreditation for each level of service provided: acute care, ambulatory care, rehabilitation, long-term care, home health care, and so on. Within each phase of care provided, emphasis is placed on staying healthy, and on preventive, curative, palliative, and end-of-life care.

Accreditation costs vary. As mentioned in Chapter 8, according to Meldi, Rhoades, and Gippe (2009), the average cost for the Joint Commission services is $33,000 for 3 years, the average cost for HFAP is $25,000 for 3 years, and the average annual cost for DNV services is $23,100. Accreditation program costs vary according to the requirements for number of surveyors depending on individual facility size and complexity. The leadership decides which accreditation system fits their vision, purpose, values, and resources. The leadership also may elect not to use accreditation but to use the CMS survey process instead.

The nurse executive should explore with the executive team the various accreditation options presented in the Myers Model. The accreditation program that is assessed to have the greatest potential to drive patient safety efforts and increase reliability of key processes should be selected.

DESIGN AT THE SYSTEM LEVEL—PATIENT SAFETY CULTURE

The nurse executive is a key member of the leadership team. She or he can present the research findings from the Myers Model to the leadership group, assess what might be needed within their organization, and implement strategic plans toward driving positive change. One area in this regard might be piloting the leadership WalkRounds to evaluate the effectiveness of this method to assist in building a better patient safety culture overall.

The nurse executive should have a clear understanding of organizational culture within his or her working environment. Assessments of organizational culture and unit cultures can be used to measure the effectiveness of leadership interventions that can be selected from the Myers Model for piloting.

Along with culture comes employee satisfaction. Sengin (2001). Kutney-Lee, McHugh, Sloane, Cimiotti, Flynn, Neff, Aiken (2009) studies linked nursing satisfaction with patient satisfaction. High turnover rates, lowered productivity, and disengaged nursing staff cost the organization lost productivity and potential delays in the performance of key patient processes. When one considers that almost 50 percent of hospital employees feel distanced or discontent in their current work, this area must be a priority for change. The Myers Model presents information on industries that maintain high employee satisfaction according to various measurements, and these examples are provided as role models.

VALUES, ETHICS, CARING, AND COURAGE

Nurse executives must have the right values and ethics to form a solid foundation on which to base decisions. She or he must "walk the talk." The challenge for a nurse executive to balance the need for reduced costs against the need for safe nurse staffing levels and an engaged work force requires ongoing discussions with the leadership team. These discussions should be relevant to patient care and should shape the nursing practice environment in such a manner that empowers nurses to grow professionally, to challenge assumptions and the status quo, and to encourage continual learning. Effective team leadership that also requires good communication skills and the courage to voice views that might not be popular with others is essential.

When making their selection, leaders should consider attributes congruent with motivating others to grow professionally, be compassionate and caring, and have respect for others. The workplace cannot tolerate bad behaviors. At the same time, if the workplace does not change for the better, nurses will continue to turn to unions as their solution toward creating a better work environment.

ORGANIZATIONAL STRUCTURES

The Myers Model for Patient Safety and Accreditation discusses organizational structures and the importance of alignment. Clearly, there is no perfect organizational structure. The structure selected by leadership should be based on an organizational assessment of where the organization is now and where it needs to be positioned in the future. One issue is clear: Developing the microsystem requires leadership commitment, a clear understanding of the aims of the microsystem, the environment of microsystem practice, and decentralization of authority so that interdisciplinary teams can effectively manage their patients, one patient at a time. A key decision here relates to ensuring that current information about quality and patient safety is available for the interdisciplinary team, so that continuous feedback and adjustments to the process of care provided can occur.

Project work is accomplished by cross-functional teams that depend on a leader sponsor for support. The leader sponsor is expected to break down any barriers that the team encounters, so that the improvement effort is successful. Team performance should be integrated into employee evaluations along with 360-degree evaluations from stakeholders as to how well leaders actually communicate with staff.

NURSING MODELS OF CARE

The Myers Model for Patient Safety and Accreditation emphasizes innovations in nursing care delivery models as formal structures within the organization. The common themes of the 24 models within the RWJF white paper, previously discussed, are well worth noting down again and include: nurses leading teams of interdisciplinary providers and ancillary staff, patients' self-management of their disease process, and alternative care settings such as the patient's home. Nurse executives should carefully evaluate each of these models to see which ones to develop within their own organization.

TEAM DEVELOPMENT AT THE MICROSYSTEMS AND EXECUTIVE LEVEL

The Myers Model for Patient Safety and Accreditation emphasizes team development at two levels: the system level and the unit level (microsystem). Hospital organizations are discovering that staff do not have effective communication skills. The hierarchies and group status of some professionals also created barriers to staff speaking up when encountering potentially unsafe behavior. Team training is recommended along with measurements to gauge the effectiveness of the training. The Team STEPPS training is one such program that may assist with increasing situational awareness and open communication at the microsystem level. (For more information on Team STEPPS, see Chapter 11.)

At the executive level, the Myers Model recommends that nurse leaders ensure that the leadership group is functioning as a team, including effective dialogue between all members of the team.

Communication skills are acquired as well. Feedback mechanisms are also needed to ensure that leadership role models the behaviors they wish to find more commonly at the microsystem level. If there is dysfunctional behavior at the top, that behavior will diffuse throughout the system and will produce poorer results than would be possible otherwise.

Another way in which the Myers Model can be helpful is for nurse executives to use it to assess health care organizations where they might want to work. The nurse executive should carefully assess if the leadership team is a "good fit" for his or her ethics/values and leadership style. Exploring the history of past nurse executives in this regard may prove useful as well.

DESIGN AT THE MICROSYSTEM LEVEL

Nurse executives should use the Myers Model to build clinical microsystems whose aim is to provide safe, effective, timely, efficient, equitable, and patient-centered care. As discussed earlier, research conducted by the RWJF found that the most effective organizations develop microsystems that focus on enterprise results, whose success can be measured (how you know the change was an improvement). Also, there needs to be motivational incentives, that are supported by an information system, and decentralize accountability at the microsystem level.

The Baldrige Model seems to be congruent with microsystem success characteristics and is also used extensively in health care to align systems toward achieving excellence in health care.

DEVELOPMENT OF A CULTURE OF SAFETY
AT THE UNIT (MICROSYSTEM) LEVEL

It is up to the nurse executive to assist in reshaping the culture from one of blaming the individual who made an honest mistake to correcting the system issues that contributed to the mistake. The AHRQ survey of 2009, which reported that only 44 percent of staff felt that their mistakes and event reports were not held against them or maintained in personnel files, shows that there is still a good deal of room for improvement in this area.

Using tools such as FMEA provides a proactive approach in designing safer systems in which care is provided. Root cause analysis enables the event to be analyzed (in a manner similar to a case study approach) and contributing causes to be corrected. Aggregate root cause analysis has the potential to identify patterns of contributing causes for corrective actions.

Nurse executives must have ongoing dialogue with the medical staff. Yet physicians, who are quite influential in shaping the culture in which care is provided, are not used to working in teams. Also, nurse executives must be effective communicators. They need to be a visible presence in the organization, so that they can role model the behaviors they wish for staff to exhibit.

As described in Chapter 10, Kalish and Begeny's I-Opt assessments, which measure information processing preferences, concluded that nurse managers will encounter layers of resistance to change within the various groups on their units, including unit secretaries and nurse aides. Nurse managers need to be taught how to manage change efforts when others think differently than they think.

Nurse executives need to ensure that all nursing staff are supported when potentially or actual unsafe behaviors are witnessed by them. The culture must be created where patients, not egos, are the priority.

DESIGN AT THE INDIVIDUAL LEVEL

The Myers Model presents evidence for the nurse executives to assess and decide on future actions. Nursing staff at the unit level should be assured of an environment that is safe, effective, timely, efficient, equitable, and patient centered. Every employee contributes to the type of culture that is experienced by patients and other staff members. In the past, health care workers would make excuses for bad behavior, such as saying things like, "He is a good surgeon. He just can't communicate well," or "That's just her personality; she doesn't mean anything by it." There should be zero tolerance for bad behavior. Nonproductive nursing time must be factored in for working and leading teams and critically analyzing nursing problems using EBP. Mentors need to be available so that nurses can challenge the old "that's the way we do things around here" mentality.

Performance evaluations should include the nurses' ability to lead and be a member of interdisciplinary teams. Nurse executives can use the Myers Model to assess their current system design at the individual level and assess for potential areas for improvement.

To increase socialization, the leaders may decide to have areas on nursing units that are shared break rooms for physicians, nurses, and other team members, and consider other design elements that foster the potential for creating and sustaining positive relationships in the work environment.

PATIENT CENTERED OR EMPLOYEE CENTERED

Nurse executives should assess what the dissatisfiers are for their nursing staff. If staffing ratios are one of them, then the nurse executive should not try to solve this problem alone. The Myers Model emphasizes that teamwork starts at the top. The executive team should do an assessment based on time-and-motion studies for nonnursing tasks that the nurses are performing and see if opportunities are present to shift these tasks to less costly workers. Also, there is the opportunity to use Lean tools to make some of the work-flow processes more efficient.

Assessment of how nurses spend their time in the health care organization is essential for seeking opportunities to improve and provide more efficient care. Documentation processes are an area to explore for opportunities to streamline the requirements and increase nursing time at the bedside. A study conducted by Tucker and Edmondson (2002) highlighted that nurses solve problems to get through a shift but do not document them as opportunities for improving efficiencies. Rather, nurses continue to do work-arounds to accomplish the required care within a set time frame. This means that the nurse executive should assess the areas in which nurses do the most "quick fixes" during a shift and take actions so that nurses don't waste time trying to solve broken processes.

Models such as Planetree have to be explored when they exceed the HCAHPS in all of the 10 measured domains in patient satisfaction. Common themes in the Planetree model include supportive and caring human interactions, social support, access to information, a healing environment, food and nutrition, arts and entertainment, human touch, and healthy communities.

As nurse executives, they must make the decision whether to embark on the Magnet journey that may enhance safe and professional nursing practice. Magnet hospitals have increased the use of certified registered nurses and maintained or increased total registered nurses hours. The Myers Model emphasizes nursing leadership's critical role in shaping the professional practice environment for nurses.

Nurse executives can influence the nursing practice environment by ensuring that nurses challenge the status quo, use evidence-based practice, and are actively engaged in shaping practice at the microsystem level. This means increased decentralization and increased empowerment for nurses working on the front line of care.

OUTCOMES

There needs to be ongoing measurement of culture, job satisfaction, preventable deaths, and adverse events to assess the effectiveness of interventions for patient safety.

CONCLUSION

The Myers Model for Patient Safety and Accreditation provides current research for nurse executives and their team to assess and make decisions for the future about their organizational architecture. The three domains of design—at the system level, the unit (microsystem) level, and individual level—all need to be in alignment with the aim of the system to provide safe, effective, timely, efficient, equitable, and patient- and employee-centered care.

REFERENCE

Meldi, D., Rhoades, F., & Gippe, A. (2009). The big three: A side by side matrix comparing hospital accrediting agencies. *Synergy, Jan/Feb*, pp. 12–14.

Sengin, K. K. (2001). The relationship between job satisfaction of registered nurses and patient satisfaction with nursing care in acute care hospitals. Dissertation Paper U of Penn. Retrieved October 20, 2011 from http://repository.upenn.edu/dissertations/AAI3003692/

Kutney-Lee, A., McHugh, M. D., Sloane, D. M., Cimiotti, J. P., Flynn, L., Neff. D. F., Airken. L. H. (2009). Nursing: A key to patient satisfaction. *Health Affairs*. July/August 28(4). 669–77

Tucker, A. L., Edmondson, A. C. (2002). Why hospitals don't learn from failures: Organizational and psychological dynamics that inhibit change. Retrieved October 20, from http://www.hbs.edu/research/facpubs/workingpapers/papers2/0203/03-059.pdf

13

Measurements and Data Integration

*I*nformation is essential to making effective decisions. The Myers Model for Patient Safety and Accreditation emphasizes information as an essential element because, without information, the organization would be running like a sailboat without a rudder, left to the mercy of the water's currents taking the organization to unknown, and most likely undesirable, destinations.

In *Alice in Wonderland*, Alice has a conversation with the Cheshire cat after she has fallen down the rabbit hole, which goes like this (Khurana, n.d.):

"Which road do I take?" said Alice.

"That depends a good deal on where you want to get to," said the Cat.

"I don't care where," said Alice.

"Then it doesn't matter which way you go," said the Cat.

The purpose of developing standardized reporting systems is to make health care systems safer by designing and/or redesigning processes to reduce or eliminate the risk of harm to patients.

Near misses and adverse events are defined and reported in many ways, which makes comparisons virtually impossible. As a result, there were and are many health care professionals who have worked to establish a standardized taxonomy to collect, aggregate, and compare patient safety events for sharing information and learning across

249

various types of health care settings. Let us recall that taxonomy is a method of classification that includes nomenclatures and hierarchical classification rules to build established relationships.

Kohn, Corrigan, and Donaldson (2000) in *To Err Is Human* addressed the issue of error-reporting systems. They reported that the Committee on Quality of Healthcare in America stated its belief that both voluntary and mandatory reporting systems are essential but should be managed separately. The committee recommended that voluntary reporting systems focus on near miss events or events that cause minimal patient harm, and that mandatory reporting systems focus on preventable adverse events (those that result in serious patient harm or death). The NQF was designated as the entity responsible for disseminating and maintaining a core set or reporting standards to be used by states. This included nomenclature and taxonomy for reporting. All health care organizations would be required to report standardized information on a defined list of adverse events.

Chang, Schyve, Croteau, O'Leary, and Loeb (2005) published the *JCAHO Patient Safety Event Taxonomy* in an attempt to standardize terminology and classification methods for near misses and adverse events. JCAHO described the following desirable attributes of the patient safety event taxonomy:

- The taxonomy would be based on clear and generally-agreed-upon terminologies and classifications.
- The taxonomy would be useful for analyzing processes and outcomes that are buried beneath the event, including the root causes and the contributing factors for the event.
- The taxonomy would facilitate a consistent collection and analysis of near miss and adverse event data across the continuum of health care systems.
- The taxonomy would be convenient and would assist with sharing and exchange of patient safety information.
- The taxonomy would be useful to assist with identifying priorities for remedial work as well as identifying the opportunities for improvement.
- The analytical framework of the model includes causes, type of errors/failures, the impact of those failures (degree of harm), and the domains in which the event occurred (settings, staff, and target).

In 2006, the WHO, World Alliance for Patient Safety Project also published a patient safety taxonomy. It defined a patient safety event as "a process or act of omission or commission that resulted in hazardous health care conditions and/or unintended harm to the patient."

An event is identified by a generalized high-level, discrete, auditable term or group of terms. The terms have good face validity. The classification scheme was designed to capture both near misses and adverse events. The conceptual framework consisted of 10 top-level classes:

1. *The event type:* Classification of the types of patient safety events that result from an omission or commission that resulted in hazardous health care conditions and/or unintended harm to the patient (e.g., falls, medication errors, clinical care, and nutrition).
2. *Contributing factors to the event:* Factors that play a part in the occurrence of a patient safety event.
3. *The event characteristics:* Contextual features surrounding the patient safety event (the type of setting, the type of staff involved, equipment involved, time of day, etc.).
4. *The patient characteristics:* the patient demographics, original reason for seeking care, and the patient's primary diagnosis
5. *The preventive factors:* Actions taken in advance to prevent the occurrence of a patient safety event (e.g., reducing overtime hours and providing adequate numbers of registered nurses in staffing ratios).
6. *The recovery factors:* Actions taken to stop circumstances or influences that lead to a patient safety event.
7. *The mitigating factors:* Factors that play a role in diminishing the impact of a patient safety event (e.g., early recognition and team communication protocols).
8. *The patient impact:* Patient outcomes (e.g., functional, physiologic, and psychologic).
9. *The organizational impact and outcomes:* The impact of organization design (e.g., legal, media, and community reputation).
10. *The actions taken:* Actions by various levels within the organization to reduce, manage, or control the harm or the likelihood of harm associated with the event. Actions may be directed at the patient level, the staff level, and/or the organizational level.

The National Quality Forum (NQF) identified patient safety taxonomy as an essential tool when implementing patient safety programs. NQF (2006) presented four consensus statements that supported the application of the *Joint Commission's Patient Safety Event Taxonomy (PSET)* as the standardized framework for classifying patient safety events. Patient safety events are classified into five areas:

1. *Impact:* Outcomes or effects of medical error and systems failure (type of patient harm).
2. *Type:* Implied or obvious visible processes that were faulty or failed.
3. *Domain:* Characteristics of the setting in which an incident occurred and the type of individuals who were involved.
4. *Cause:* Factors and agents that led to the incident that occurred.
5. *Prevention and mitigation:* Measures that were taken or proposed to reduce the incidence and effects of adverse occurrences.

NQF recommended that federal agencies such as the U.S. DHHS, the Department of Veterans Affairs, the Department of Defense, and others include patient safety taxonomy as part of the national health information standards, which are spread to others by them.

The Joint Commission was charged with the ongoing maintenance, testing, and evolution of the database as needed, working with the various users.

WHO's Alliance for Patient Safety (n.d.) introduced the taxonomy to facilitate improved information sharing for learning and exchange of information to reduce health care–related harm. The drafting group made a critical decision to build on the previous work done by Joint Commission's Patient Safety Event Taxonomy, which was endorsed by the NQF in the United States as well as by other agencies globally.

The taxonomy is free and can be downloaded at www.who.int/patientsafety/taxonomy/evolution/en/index.html.

The Joint Commission was awarded a contract by the WHO to provide oversight for the global field-testing of the International Classification for Patient Safety (ICPS) (BNET, 2007).

American Society for Healthcare Risk Management is a personal membership group of the AHA whose members represent health care, insurance, law, and other related professions. ASHRM focuses on developing and implementing safe and effective patient care practices across all health care settings.

ASHRM (2008) published a monograph that emphasized the importance of having a patient safety taxonomy and evaluated the existing patient safety taxonomies. ASHRM recommended that risk managers consider the following when implementing a reporting system for medical events:

■ Ensure that the taxonomy selected include existing and proposed classification models that are well known, available, and widely accepted.

■ Ensure that the taxonomy selected meets the regulatory and statu-
tory requirements for the reporting of patient safety events.

■ Ensure that the taxonomy is designed in a manner that provides
data-driven decision support. It needs to be easy for clinicians and
business decision makers to use. The taxonomy should be easy to
read, and the data mining capabilities need to be evaluated.

■ Ensure that the taxonomy has the capability to integrate and map
current coding systems where applicable.

■ Ensure that the taxonomy is easy to integrate with other information systems.

The PSQIA was enacted with the aim to encourage the expansion of
voluntary, provider-driven initiatives to improve the quality and safety
of health care, to promote speedier transmission of information to promote learning about the underlying causes of both the risks and harms
in health care, and to ensure that these findings are widely shared.
A copy of the Patient Safety Act is at www.pso.ahrq.gov/statute/
pl109-41.htm.

The data submitted to the PSO by provider organizations, physicians, and other clinicians will be considered privileged and confidential for use in quality and safety efforts.

PSOs are entities or components of other organizations that ensure
that certain AHRQ Safety Rule criteria are met. The primary purpose
of a PSO is to conduct patient safety activities to improve patient safety
and quality (AHRQ, 2005).

The Government Accountability Office (GAO) 2010's report stated
that there were 65 PSOs as of July 2009. Of the 17 PSOs randomly selected
for interviews, only a few of them actually had entered into contracts
to work with providers or had begun to receive any patient safety data.
Some PSOs were waiting for AHRQ to establish a standardized method
for PSOs to collect data from their providers; other PSOs were engaged
in educating their providers regarding confidentiality protections.

The AHRQ was working on the standardized formats PSOs and
providers would use when submitting patient safety data to the
NPSD along with a method for de-identifying the information. The
target date AHRQ set if progress goes as expected for NPSD to begin
receiving patient safety data from hospitals was February 2011.

AHRQ uses its published "Common Formats" to describe the
clinical nomenclature and technical requirements developed for the
standardized collection and reporting of patient safety data, including
all supporting material.

The AHRQ's Common Format Version 1.1 has a defined focus on
patient safety reporting for acute care hospitals. These reports have

privilege and confidentiality protections of the Patient Safety Act and Patient Safety Rule.

The scope of Common Formats applies to all patient safety concerns and includes patient safety events that reached the patient, whether harm to the patient occurred or not (incidents); patient safety events that did not reach the patient (near misses or close calls); and circumstances that increase the probability of a patient safety event (unsafe conditions).

The Common Formats are also aligned with the WHO concepts, framework, and definitions contained in their draft ICPS.

AHRQ Common Formats Version 1.1. is available at www.psoppc .org/web/patientsafety.

VOLUNTARY REPORTING SYSTEMS

Voluntary reporting systems can be a potential source of valuable information for patient safety improvement efforts; however, continued chronic underreporting of events is extensive. The GAO (2000) cited the common reasons for underreporting as fear of being blamed, the fear of being sued, and an expectation that reporting will not help anything anyway. Also, there might be confusion on what is reported due to ambiguity in the definition of adverse events. The GAO concluded that even with the limitations of underreporting, valuable information could still be generated to help in reducing medical errors.

Voluntary reporting systems may be managed at either the institutional level or at the government level. These systems assist with the identification of system vulnerabilities. These should include near misses, also called close calls, and any hazardous situation, which if left unchanged could potentially lead to an undesirable outcome. Voluntary reporting systems need to have funding and legislative protections so that users of the system will not be afraid to report for the fear of legal actions that might arise against them.

INSTITUTE FOR SAFE MEDICATION PRACTICES

The Institute for Safe Medicine Practices (ISMP) (n.d.) operates the Medication Error Reporting Program (MERP) in cooperation with the United States Pharmacopoeia (USP). The information obtained is fed back to the institutions through ISMP's initiatives to improve the medication use process, and directly impacts both product and clinician practice changes. This is a confidential, national reporting system and offers legal protection as a federally certified PSO. When there is a concern for safety, the information is shared with the Food and Drug Administration (FDA) Med Watch reporting program to expedite necessary changes.

Some examples of the impact of the ISMP (MERP) include:

- Numerous nationwide hazard alerts have been widely reported. Some examples include reports on the fatal events involving concentrated electrolytes in 1996, fatal events involving magnesium sulfate overdoses in 1997, and methotrexate overdoses in 2002 due to the physician ordering administration daily instead of weekly.
- ISMP is working with others to establish guidelines, standards, and goals such as when ISMP's campaign influenced the Veterans Administration and the Joint Commission to require removal of concentrated potassium chloride for injection from all patient care units in 1997.
- ISMP has several advocacy initiatives such as holding the first Global Conference on MERP. Approximately 100 pharmacists from around the world attended this program.

For a complete list of ISMP's accomplishments go to: www.ismp .org/about/merpimpact.asp.

ISMP is the only nonprofit organization in the United States devoted to medication error prevention and safe medication use. Information is collected for errors, near misses, or hazardous conditions, which include and are not limited to administering the wrong drug, dose, or strength, confusion over drugs which look alike or sound alike, preparation or calculation errors, misuse of medical equipment, incorrect route of administration of drug, and any errors in the process of medications related to prescribing, transcribing, dispensing, or monitoring. Providing identification information of the reporter is optional. An electronic form is available on the ISMP website at www.ismp.org/orderforms/reporterrortoismp.asp.

SENTINEL EVENTS DATABASE

The Joint Commission established its SEs policy in 1996 for accredited organizations. A SE is defined as "an unexpected occurrence involving death or serious physical or psychological injury, or the risk thereof. Serious injury specifically includes loss of limb or function. The phrase 'or the risk thereof' includes any process variation for which a recurrence would carry a significant chance of a serious adverse outcome. Such events are called 'sentinel' because they signal the need for immediate investigation and response."

Accredited organizations are expected to identify and respond to SEs in a manner that will significantly reduce and/or eliminate the likelihood of the adverse event from occurring again. The process that is implemented for accomplishing this aim is the RCA process. RCA focuses on systems, not staff, and progresses from the sharp end (special cause) to the blunt end (common causes). Action plans include effectiveness measures and timelines for accomplishing the objectives.

The Joint Commission maintains a Sentinel Events Database and issues Sentinel Events Alerts. Wrong-site surgeries continued to be at the top of the list for types of SEs in 2010. Communication failures accounted for more than 60 percent of the root causes for SEs in 2007 (see Table 13.1). The Joint Commission responded to this information by including effective communication as one of its NPSG (Roberts, 2007).

Joint Commission, www.jointcommission.org/SentinelEvents/Statistics/

TABLE 13.1
Joint Commission Sentinel Events Database

Total Number of SEs Reviewed by The Joint Commission Since January 1995	6782	
TYPE OF SE	#	%
Wrong-site surgery	908	13.4
Suicide	804	11.9
Op/post-op complication	734	10.8
Delay in treatment	580	8.6
Medication error	547	8.1
Patient fall	436	6.4
Unintended retention of foreign body*	360	5.3
Assault/rape/homicide	256	3.8
Perinatal death/loss of function	209	3.1
Patient death/injury in restraints	201	3.0
Transfusion error	146	2.2
Infection-related event	145	2.1

TABLE 13.1 (*continued*)

TYPE OF SE	#	%
Medical equipment-related	135	2.0
Fire	102	1.5
Anesthesia-related event	100	1.5
Patient elopement	99	1.5
Maternal death	94	1.4
Ventilator death/injury	62	0.9
Abduction	32	0.5
Utility systems-related event	25	0.4
Infant discharge to wrong family	8	0.1
†Other less frequent types	799	11.8

SELF-REPORTED SEs BY YEAR	# NON-SELF-REPORTED	# SELF-REPORTED	% SELF-REPORTED
1995	22	1	4
1996	31	3	9
1997	123	16	12
1998	50	130	72
1999	55	278	83
2000	87	270	76
2001	101	336	77
2002	146	269	65
2003	174	313	64
2004	214	347	62
2005	215	367	63
2006	182	344	65
2007	293	450	61
2008	305	510	63
2009	344	624	64
2010 1st Q	60	122	67

METHOD FOR REVIEW OF HCO RESPONSE TO SE	#	%
Alternative 0 RCA submitted to Joint Commission	5194	76.6
Alternative 1 RCA brought to Central office	1097	16.2

(*continued*)

TABLE 13.1 (*continued*)

METHOD FOR REVIEW OF HCO RESPONSE TO SE	#	%
Alternative 2 RCA documents reviewed on-site	171	2.5
Alternative 3 RCA reviewed by interviews on-site	217	3.2
Alternative 4 Responses inferred from process; P&P	103	1.5

SE SETTING	#	%
Hospital	4590	67.7
Psychiatric hospital	734	10.8
Psych unit in general hospital	332	4.9
Behavioral health facility	299	4.4
Emergency department	298	4.4
Ambulatory care	203	3.0
Long term care facility	160	2.4
Home care	126	1.9
Office-based surgery	20	0.3
Clinical laboratory	9	0.1
Others[‡]	11	0.2

SOURCE OF SE	#	%
Self-report	4381	64.6
Complaints	1014	15.0
Identified during survey	574	8.5
Media	414	6.1
CMS or state reports	399	5.9

SE OUTCOMES	#	%
Patient death	4642	67
Loss of function	638	9
Others[§]	1640	24
Total patients impacted	6920	100

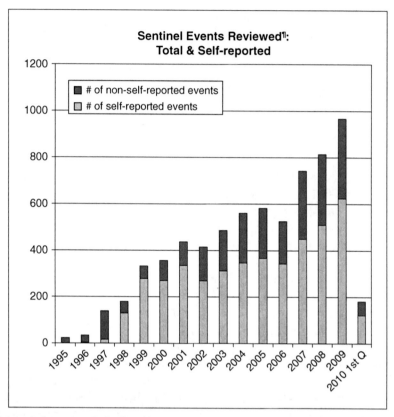

* Unintended retention of a foreign object was added to the definition of reviewable events
  June 2005. This data represents events reviewed since that date, not 1995–2009.

† Others include: Inpatient drug overdose, self-inflicted injury, severe neonatal
  hyperbilirubinemia, radiation overdose, dialysis-related event, transfer-related event,
  and other anticipated events.

‡ Other includes: Disease specific care, diagnostic imaging, hospice care.

§ Other includes: Unexpected additional care/extended care, and psychological impact.

¶ This graph represents all RCAs reviewed and accepted in a particular calendar year.

(© The Joint Commission, 2010. Reprinted with permission.)

PATIENT SAFETY REPORTING SYSTEM

The Patient Safety Reporting System (PSRS) is a nonpunitive, confidential, voluntary reporting system in which staff can report near misses, incident- and event-related information and data with the aim to improve patient safety. PSRS is managed by NASA. It is open for use to any medical systems, and reporters can submit PSRS reports directly to NASA by electronic forms or via the U.S. mail.

PSRS is meant to be complementary to the medical organization's internal reporting system. It removes identification from reports before they are entered into the incident database.

The PSRS form for reporting can be downloaded at www.psrs.arc .nasa.gov/reportingform/downloadform.html.

MEDMARX®

MEDMARX was managed by USP until December 2008. Until that time, from 2001 to 2008, USP analyzed medication error reports submitted by facilities participating in its national medication error and adverse drug reactions reporting program. From this information, the following reports were compiled and shared (USP, n.d.).

- Mandatory External Reporting
- State Adverse Event Reporting
- In December 2008, the GAO issued a report *Adverse Events in Hospitals—State Reporting Systems.*

Key results included the following:

As of January 2008, there were 26 states that had hospital adverse event reporting systems, 10 of which had been operational for less than 3 years, and one other state had taken action to develop one. All of the states that reported had state laws in place that authorized the systems, had formal policies and procedures in place for reporting, and were actively collecting data from hospitals.

The types of events reported, the criteria used to determine what events would be reported, and the type of information reported varied widely. The state criteria for determining if an event was to be reported focused on the degree of harm experienced by the patient. Each of the 26 state systems had different requirements regarding the information that had to be included with the event.

Staff from 15 of the 26 states acknowledged underreporting to the state reporting systems. Twenty-three states reported using the data received to hold individual hospitals accountable; 18 also reported that the data were used to promote learning and prevent adverse events. Adverse event reports resulted in desk or on-site audits, and/or state-led investigations of the hospitals' handling of the reported events. Four of these states also reported that this information was used in licensing decisions for hospitals.

The key conclusions from this report centered around the wide variations that make the reporting system unsuitable for identifying any national incidence and trends.

Centers for Disease Control and Prevention (CDC)—National Nosocomial Infections Surveillance System (NNIS)

History: The NNIS system report was established in 1970 and has been serving as an aggregation system for more than 30 years.

Role/Reports: NNIS is a voluntary reporting system that was established to monitor hospital-acquired infections, and provides guidance on prevention efforts to infection control practitioners. Data are collected using standardized protocols. The classifications system includes categories for major and specific infection sites using uniform CDC definitions that include laboratory and clinical criteria (NNIS, 2004).

Website: www.cdc.gov/ncidod/dhqp

Dialysis Surveillance Network

History: The Dialysis Surveillance Network is a voluntary national surveillance system initiated by the CDC in 1999 to assist hemodialysis centers in tracking vascular access infections and other bacterial infections in dialysis patients. It also monitors the rates of colonization and infection by antimicrobial resistant bacteria in these patients.

Role/Reports: The data gathered are used to compare rates between participating centers for benchmarking and to assist with motivation changes in practices among the centers, to prevent further infections.

Website: www.cdc.gov/ncidod/dhqp

Mandatory Reporting Systems

1. FDA
   a. *History*: The FDA is the oldest consumer protection agency in the U.S. federal government. Its regulatory functions began with the passage of the 1906 Pure Food and Drugs Act, which provided consumers basic elements of protection that protected against misbranded and adulterated food and drugs.

b. *Role/Reports*: The FDA is responsible for protection of the public by ensuring the safety, efficacy, and security of human and veterinary drugs, biological products, medical devices, cosmetics, and any products that emit radiation. Med Watch is the FDA's safety information and adverse event reporting program. It contains both voluntary and mandatory reporting systems.

c. *Website*: www.fda.gov/default.htm

2. OSHA

a. *History*: The OSHA of 1970 was the first of public efforts to provide protection to workers from harm on the job. This act established a federal, national program to protect the entire workforce from injury or death occurring in the workplace (MacLaury, 1984).

b. *Role/Reports*: OSHA requires employers with 11 or more employees to maintain injury and illness reports. The employer must complete two forms; one known as the OSHA log that itemizes each injury and illness that occurred during the year; the other form provides supplementary details about the injury or illness.

   The BLS and participating state agencies conduct an annual survey of employers in almost all sector of private industry to collect and aggregate survey results for public information and research.

c. *Website*: www.osha.gov/pls/oshaweb/owadisp.show_document? p_id=16312&p_table=FEDERAL_REGISTER

3. Vaccine Adverse Event Reporting System (VAERS)

a. *History*: The VAERS is the national vaccine safety surveillance program. It is co-sponsored by the CDC and the FDA. VAERS originated from the National Childhood Vaccine Injury Act (NCVIA) of 1986, which required health care professionals and vaccine manufacturers to report to the U.S. DHHS specific adverse events that occur after administration of routine vaccines. VAERS was started in 1990 in response to this legislation.

b. *Role/Reports*: VAERS receives approximately 30,000 reports annually, and 13 percent of them are classified as serious, which means they are associated with disability, hospitalization, life-threatening illness, or death. About 85 to 90 percent of the reports describe mild adverse reactions such as fever, local reactions, and episodes of crying or mild irritability.

   Anyone can file a VAERS report, including health care providers, manufacturers, and vaccine recipients. VAERS is a

voluntary reporting system except when the adverse event qualifies under the criteria for "reportable events." An example of a
reportable event would be the patient experiencing anaphylaxis
or anaphylactic shock within 7 days of receiving a hepatitis B
vaccine.

   c. *Website*: http://vaers.hhs.gov/index/about/index

Standardized nomenclature for patient safety in which to build reporting systems is necessary in health care. The standardized nomenclature
needs to integrate all types of errors so that patterns can be seen easily.

   Isolated reports obscure patterns and prevent learning from occurring. A patient safety culture demands that information be optimized
to enhance learning opportunities that expose and mitigate or eliminate risk to patients.

   Reporting systems at the national level are still under development. Health care organizations should use a taxonomy when
classifying patient safety events. It should be congruent with external
reporting systems as they continue to be developed.

REFERENCES

AHRQ. (2005). *Patient safety and quality improvement act of 2005.* Retrieved
   June 10, 2010, from http://www.pso.ahrq.gov/statute/pl109-41.htm

American Society for Healthcare Risk Management. (2008). *Tackling patient safety
   taxonomy: A must for risk managers.* ASHRM Monograph. Retrieved June 5,
   2010, from http://www.ashrm.org/ashrm/education/development/
   monographs/index.shtml

BNET. (2007, November–December). *Joint commission to test international classification for patient safety.* Retrieved June 5, 2010, from http://findarticles
   .com/p/articles/mi_m0FSW/is_6_25/ai_n24958210/?tag=content;col1

Chang, A. W., Schyve, P. M., Croteau, R. J., O'Leary, D., & Loeb, J. M. (2005).
   The JCAHO patient safety event taxonomy: a standardized terminology
   and classification schema for near misses and adverse events. *International
   Journal for Quality in Health Care, February,* pp. 1–11.

Government Accountability Office. (2008). *Adverse events in hospitals state
   reporting systems* (OEI-06-07-00471). Retrieved June 10, 2010, http://
   oig.hhs.gov/search/index.asp?submitted=submitted&q=oei-06-07-
   00471&output=xml_no_dtd&sort=date%3AD%3AL%3Ad1&ie=UTF-
   8&oe=UTF-8&lr=lang_en&client=oig&ud=1&site=oig&proxystylesheet=
   oig_test&proxyreload=1&submit=

Government Accountability Office. (2010). *Patient safety act: HHS in the process of implementing the act, so its effectiveness cannot yet be evaluated* (GAO-1-281). Retrieved June 10, 2010, from http://www.gao.gov/products/GAO-10-281

Institute for Safe Medicine Practices. (n.d.). *ISMP medication errors reporting program (MERP)*. Retrieved June 5, 2010, from https://www.ismp.org/orderforms/reporterrortoismp.asp

Khurana, S. (n.d.). *Lewis Caroll quotes: Alice in Wonderland*. Retrieved June 5, 2010, from http://quotations.about.com/od/moretypes/a/alice4.htm

Kohn, L. T., Corrigan, J. M., & Donaldson, M. S. (2000). *To err is human: Building a safer health system*. Washington, DC: National Academy Press.

MacLaury, J. (1984). *United States department of labor. The occupational safety and health administration: A history of its first thirteen years, 1971–1984*. Retrieved June 10, 2010, from http://www.dol.gov/oasam/programs/history/mono-osha13introtoc.htm

NNIS. (2004). National Nosocomial Infections Surveillance (NNIS) system report, data summary from January 1992 through June 2004, issued October, 2004. *American Journal Infection Control*. Retrieved June 10, 2010, from http://www.cdc.gov/nhsn/

National Quality Forum. (2006). *Standardizing a patient safety taxonomy: A consensus report*. NQF. http://www.psnet.ahrq.gov/resource.aspx?resourceID=3358

Roberts, D. (2007). Clear communication, accept nothing less. *Med/Surg Nursing*. June *16*(3). 142, 148.

United States General Accountability Office (GAO). (2000). *Adverse events: Surveillance systems for adverse events and medical errors* (GAO/T-HEHS-00-61). Retrieved January 30, 2011, from http://docs.google.com/viewer?a=v&q=cache:k2WINormGZ4J:www.gao.gov/archive/2000/he00061t.pdf+GAO+(2000).+Adverse+Events:+Surveillance+systems+for+adverse+events+and+medical&hl=en&gl=us&pid=bl&srcid=ADGEESgHPAhid0GFmJjVVX7BsWXjGUlu3M4iSoYhkYxiDvMJA52dIoxq90vzN_Ajh1HdYMTSwa3Gqlthv_t69jsnSMZOqFehmrTAvmo5IDIdHryzTyjhraob9JjZk9Brqw_V_YyEf4cn&sig=AHIEtbQoqy1K__4rKI3K5IWMt-k4lvhmVg

USP. (n.d.). *MEDMARX® data reports*. Retrieved June 10, 2010, from http://www.usp.org/products/medMarx/

World Health Organization. (n.d.). *International classification for patient safety*. Retrieved June 5, 2010, from http://www.who.int/patientsafety/implementation/taxonomy/

14

Root Cause Analysis and Failure Mode and Effects Analysis

*I*t is often said among nursing staff that nurses make the worst patients. They know that there is no such thing as a simple surgery; that Murphy's Law is highly applicable in health care; that "If anything can go wrong, it will go wrong"; and "If you think everything is going perfectly, then you have obviously overlooked something."

The Joint Commission has been tracking SEs for over 10 years. Wrong-site surgeries have been reported to be increasing annually since 1995, even after Universal Precautions to prevent wrong-site surgeries were implemented as a Joint Commission requirement in 2004. Why this is happening is not known; however, as the Joint Commission relies on voluntary reporting, the uptick can be due to increased reporting of these events.

AHRQ (n.d.) describes RCA as the structured method used to analyze adverse events of a serious nature.

Originally used to determine the cause of industrial accidents, RCA then found use in health care settings. The goals of an RCA are clear: to find out what happened, why and how it happened, and what can be done to reduce the likelihood of reoccurrence.

The Joint Commission requires that RCA be performed for SEs and for any occurrence that meets the following criteria: an unexpected death or major permanent loss of function that was not part of the patient's underlying condition or related to the natural course of the patient's illness.

The event can also involve:

- Suicide of any patient who received care, treatment, and services in a 24/7 staffed care setting or within 72 hours following discharge
- Unexpected death of a full-term infant
- Abduction of any patient who was receiving care, treatment, and services
- An infant who was discharged to the wrong family
- Rape
- A hemolytic transfusion reaction that involved administration of blood or blood products having major blood group incompatibilities
- Any surgery performed on the wrong patient or wrong body part
- Any surgery where there was an unintended retention of a foreign object in the patient following surgery or other invasive procedure
- Severe neonatal hyperbilirubinemia
- Fluoroscopy that was prolonged with cumulative doses greater than or equal to 1500 rads to a single field or any delivery of radiotherapy to the wrong body region or greater than 25 percent above the planned radiotherapy dosage

The RCA process involves drilling down to uncover underlying problems that contributed to the medical error without focusing on the mistakes made by the individuals involved in the case. Latent errors are generally hidden system issues that contribute to adverse events. RCA starts at the sharp end (provider level) and ends up at the blunt end (the system level).

RCAs need to have a standardized protocol that begins with timely data collection that includes the contextual features surrounding the adverse event obtained through medical record review, interviewing staff, and examining any equipment, and so on, that were associated with the adverse event.

After the data collection, a multidisciplinary team is convened. This team must understand their role and how the RCA process works. Generally, a facilitator with specialized training (e.g., patient safety officer or quality manager) is assigned for an RCA.

The Joint Commission has required RCA in accredited hospitals for over 10 years. Each analysis should be thorough and credible. To be thorough, the RCA must include the following:

1. The team needs to identify the human and other factors that were the most directly associated with the SE's occurrence along with the system's processes related to the occurrence.

2. The team needs to demonstrate an analysis that digs deeper into system issues and processes through a series of "Why?" questions.

3. The team needs to use the Joint Commission root cause matrix and include for review all areas that were appropriate to the specific type of event.

4. The team needs to identify the risk points along with their potential contributions to this type of event.

5. The team needs to determine potential improvement in processes or systems that, if implemented, would tend to decrease the likelihood of recurrence in the future, or determine after analysis that no such opportunity exists.

6. To be credible, the Joint Commission requires that:
   a. The team includes participation by the leadership and by staff who are closest to the process under review.
   b. The review be internally consistent. This means that there is no contradictory logic or that the team did not address obvious questions.
   c. There be an explanation for all findings that the team identifies as "no problem" or "not applicable."
   d. There be a literature review performed when appropriate Joint Commission (2009).

It is helpful to have ground rules for review at the first RCA team meeting (e.g., focus on systems; not people). It is also important to note that the Joint Commission has a minimum scope of RCA expected for specific types of SEs.

For example, it is expected that RCAs for medical errors include the following to determine if any qualify as a contributing cause: physical assessment process, patient identification process, care planning process, continuum of care, staffing levels, orientation and training of staff, competency assessment/credentialing, supervision of staff, communication with patient/family, communication among staff members, availability of information, adequacy of technological support, equipment maintenance/management, physical environment, and medication management as appropriate for the event.

It is also helpful to have the following information collected as soon as possible after the event: interviews, working schedules, medical record review, equipment examination, policies and procedures, and literature review when appropriate.

Events that are not recommended for RCA include events that are the result of a criminal act, a purposefully unsafe act where the provider intended to cause harm by his or her actions, acts that are related to substance abuse by provider staff, and events involving suspected patient abuse of any kind. These four types of events should be referred to administration for disciplinary or administrative action (Canadian Patient Safety Institute, 2006).

A narrative description of the event, followed by the team's initial flow chart of the sequence of events, also assists with further drilldown for examining what happened then comparing to what should have happened, and exploring why it happened.

Flow charts provide a visual display of the sequence of events that led to the adverse event and also provide a visual display of what should have happened under normal circumstances. Comparing the two flow charts makes it easier for the team to identify undesirable variation, waiting times, and risk points.

One tool used widely for RCA is the fishbone diagram. It is broken into subcategories that continue to be broken down and detailed through the series of "why" questions.

Barrier analysis involves the analysis of equipment, design, administrative and work processes, supervisory and management, knowledge and skills, and physical and warning devices that were deficient in preventing the event. A systematic review of what the barriers are and why they failed in this event is helpful to identify the causal factors of the adverse event.

Causal statements are developed from the final flow chart and why it occurred, and contributing factor(s) statements are developed for each failed process. For example: "The absence of a clear procedure that outlined each nurse's role in double-checking the high-risk medication increased the likelihood that the insulin dosage was not correct." There are rules for causal statements. A copy of the rules for causal statements adopted from David Marx, can be obtained from the National Center for Patient Safety (NCPS) at http://www.patientsafety .gov/glossary.html

Actions for the organization depend on the type of risk identified and the feasibility for implementation. Actions can be control of the risk, elimination of the risk, or acknowledgment and acceptance of the risk. For example, in reference to number 5 above, when seeking to control the risk, revise the procedure for double-checking high-risk medications by nursing staff, so that each nurse knows his or her role and performs it on a consistent basis. Or, when seeking to control the risk to patients associated with available concentrated electrolytes stored on the nursing unit, consider removing those electrolytes from the nursing units altogether; resulting in no possibility for patient harm.

The organization may choose to accept the risk if the action to counter it completely is not currently feasible while implementing a weaker measure of control. For example, the hospital cannot implement CPOE this year; however, it is budgeted for next year. Until then, the hospital places several measures into effect in an attempt to control the risk: double checks of high-risk medications, elimination of prohibited abbreviations, standardized drips, mini-software programs for high-risk medications such as chemotherapy, and so on.

The implementation plan is accompanied by measures of effectiveness that determine not just the completion but the effectiveness of the action. Measures of success (MOS) are numerical or quantifiable measures based on an audit with an adequate sample size that evaluates if the planned action chosen was effective and sustainable.

The Joint Commission requires MOS compliance percentages to be 90 or 100 percent depending on the identified association to the elements of performance to standards or NPS goals. If actions cannot be associated with standards or NPS goals, then the level of compliance must be 85 percent, and requires the Joint Commission approval.

There are stringent reporting requirements for MOS by the Joint Commission. If health care organizations do not comply, their status may change from Accreditation to Conditional Accreditation as a penalty (Joint Commission, 2009).

Latent errors are embedded in the layers of the system that contributed to the medical error. There are many contributing factors that have led to latent errors. AHRQ categorizes latent errors into the following areas:

- *Staffing*: A nurse who works a lot of mandatory overtime hours miscalculates the dosage and the patient receives four times the normal dose of heparin, resulting in a GI bleed that requires 10 units of blood.

- *Organizational*: A nurse does not report her medication error because of the fear of being punished by the management; as a result of her error, the patient gets a central line infection that results in 10 days' additional hospital stay for antibiotic therapy.
- *Task-related*: A new graduate nurse miscalculates an insulin dose, which results in the patient being treated for severe hypoglycemia.
- *Team environment*: The surgeon ignores the team and states that the time-out process is stupid and asks to continue without it. As a result, the patient has surgery on the wrong body part.
- *Work environment*: Every unit has a different brand of IV pump due to an attempt for the hospital to reduce costs; the IV pumps have not been standardized. A nurse is floated to another unit to work and makes a mistake using an IV pump she is unfamiliar with and the patient receives 10 times the normal dosage of a medication resulting in the patient experiencing a respiratory arrest with transfer to IC.
- *Institutional/regulatory*: Hospital administration is putting pressure on the staff to open a new service without adequate nurse staffing. The patient-to-nurse ratio is 9 patients to 1 nurse and the patient experiences a cardiac arrest due to failure to rescue.
- *Patient characteristics*: The patient has poor vision and miscalculates his insulin dosage, resulting in severe hypoglycemic shock.

Even though RCA is widely used and is a requirement by the Joint Commission for SEs, there is a paucity of research to support its effectiveness in health care. When RCA is performed, it is from one single case study; therefore, it may prevent another adverse event only when the alignment of events occurs in the same sequence as in the case under study (AHRQ, n.d.).

AHRQ reported that the problem is not in the performance of the RCA, but in the analysis and follow-up for the RCA. Also, there is not a standardized method for aggregation of RCAs with their analysis performed at various organizations so that patterns can be analyzed to recommend solutions.

Many states do require that RCAs be reported to them after serious events occur.

There are numerous tools and implementation manuals for performing an RCA. Some of the better-known information comes from the following websites free of charge:

1. www.nrls.npsa.nhs.uk/resources/?q=0+rca NPSA in the UK: Contains numerous templates, investigational tools, RCA investigation with triggers, and a guide for aggregated and multi-incident RCA investigations.
2. www.patientsafetyinstitute.ca/English/toolsResources/rca/ Documents/March%202006%20RCA%20Workbook.pdf Canadian RCA Framework: A tool for identifying and addressing the root causes of critical incidents in health care. Produced by the CPSI and the ISMP Canada.
3. www.patientsafety.gov/CogAids/RCA/index.html#page=page-1 United States Department of Veterans Affairs: NCPS: Contains definitions, diagrams, and step-by-step instructions on how to perform an RCA.
4. www.JointCommission.org/SentinelEvents/Forms/ The Joint Commission has SE forms and tools along with sample policies and their matrix for RCA at this website.

The Joint Commission's framework for conducting an RCA and action plan includes a template to aid the team in going through the steps of the RCA process (see Table 14.1).

FAILURE MODE AND EFFECTS ANALYSIS (FMEA)

RCA digs deeper into the roots of the system after the event has occurred. Essentially, RCA analyzes a case study retrospectively; FMEA analyzes a process prospectively.

FMEA is a proactive method to determine the reliability and the effect of system and equipment failures if they occur.

Each failure mode is classified by its severity to determine the effect of failures on the system. This process identifies the system vulnerabilities; consequently, actions can be taken to prevent adverse events from occurring. Some comparisons of FMEA and RCA are shown in Table 14.2.

FMEA is process focused. The vulnerabilities of process are analyzed. RCA looks at all the reasons why an event occurred. FMEA is prospective. It is preventive in nature and also proactive because processes are studied to analyze the system design to identify and deal with vulnerabilities.

TABLE 14.1

A Framework for a Root Cause Analysis and Action Plan in Response to a SE

LEVEL OF ANALYSIS	QUESTIONS	FINDINGS	ROOT CAUSE?	ASK "WHY?"	TAKE ACTION
What happened?					
SE	What are the details of the event? (Brief description)				
	When did the event occur? (Date, day of week, time)				
	What area/service was impacted?				
Why did it happen?					
The process or activity in which the event occurred.	What are the steps in the process, as designed? (A flow diagram may be helpful here.)				
What were the most proximate factors?	What steps were involved in (contributed to) the event?				
(Typically "special cause" variation)					
Human factors	What human factors were relevant to the outcome?				
Equipment factors	How did the equipment performance affect the outcome?				
Controllable environmental factors	What factors directly affected the outcome?				
Uncontrollable external factors	Are they truly beyond the organization's control?				
Others	Are there any other factors that have directly influenced this outcome?				
	What other areas or services are impacted?				

Reprinted with permission from ©Joint Commission: Framework for conducting a root cause analysis.

This template is provided as an aid in organizing the steps in a root cause analysis. Not all possibilities and questions will apply in every case, and there may be others that will emerge in the course of the analysis. However, all possibilities and questions should be fully considered in your quest for root cause and risk reduction.

As an aid to avoiding "loose ends," the three columns on the right are provided to be checked off for later reference:

■ "Root cause?" should be answered "yes" or "no" for each finding. A root cause is typically a finding related to a process or system that has a potential for redesign to reduce risk. If a particular finding that is relevant to the event is not a root cause, be sure that it is addressed later in the analysis with a "Why?" question. Each finding that is identified as a root cause should be considered for an action and addressed in the action plan.

■ "Ask 'why?'" should be checked off whenever it is reasonable to ask why the particular finding occurred (or didn't occur when it should have)—in other words, to drill down further. Each item checked in this column should be addressed later in the analysis with a "why?" question. It is expected that any significant findings that are not identified as root causes themselves have "roots."

■ "Take action?" should be checked for any finding that can reasonably be considered for a risk reduction strategy. Each item checked in this column should be addressed later in the action plan. It will be helpful to write the number of the associated action item in the "Take action?" column for each of the findings that requires an action.

Why did that happen? What systems and processes underlie those proximate factors?	Human resources issues	To what degree are staff properly qualified and currently competent for their responsibilities?
(Common cause variation here may lead to special cause variation in dependent processes)		How did actual staffing compare with ideal levels?

(continued)

page 2 of 4

TABLE 14.1 (*Continued*)

LEVEL OF ANALYSIS	QUESTIONS	FINDINGS	ROOT CAUSE?	ASK "WHY?"	TAKE ACTION
	What are the plans for dealing with contingencies that would tend to reduce effective staffing levels?				
	To what degree is staff performance in the operant process(es) addressed?				
	How can orientation and inservice training be improved?				
Information management issues	To what degree is all necessary information available when needed? Accurate? Complete? Unambiguous?				
	To what degree is communication among participants adequate?				
Environmental management issues	To what degree is the physical environment appropriate for the processes being carried out?				
	What systems are in place to identify environmental risks?				
	What emergency and failure-mode responses have been planned and tested?				
Leadership issues: – Corporate culture	To what degree is the culture conducive to risk identification and reduction?				
– Encouragement of communication	What are the barriers to communication of potential risk factors?				
– Clear communication of priorities	To what degree is the prevention of adverse outcomes communicated as a high priority? How?				
– Uncontrollable factors	What can be done to protect against the effects of these uncontrollable factors?				

Reprinted with permission from ©Joint Commission: Framework for conducting a root cause analysis.

ACTION PLAN	RISK REDUCTION STRATEGIES	MEASURES OF EFFECTIVENESS
For each of the findings identified in the analysis as requiring an action, indicate the planned action expected, implementation date, and associated measure of effectiveness. OR . . .	**Action Item #1:**	
If after consideration of such a finding a decision is made not to implement an associated risk reduction strategy, indicate the rationale for not taking action at this time.	**Action Item #2:**	
Check to be sure that the selected measure will provide data that will permit assessment of the effectiveness of the action.	**Action Item #3:**	
Consider whether pilot testing of a planned improvement should be conducted.	**Action Item #4:**	
Improvements to reduce risk should ultimately be implemented in all areas where applicable, not just where the event occurred. Identify where the improvements will be implemented.	**Action Item #5:**	
	Action Item #6:	
	Action Item #7:	
	Action Item #8:	

Cite any books or journal articles that were considered in developing this analysis and action plan:

Reprinted with permission from ©Joint Commission: Framework for conducting a root cause analysis.

According to Stalhandske, De Rosier, Wilson, and Murphy (2009), in 1949 there was a military manual titled *Procedure for Performing a Failure Mode, Effects and Analysis.*

The failures were classified according to their impact on the success of the mission and personnel and equipment safety. This process was subsequently adopted by the NASA and used for tests on missions such as Apollo. Later, FMEA was used in automobile manufacturing and finally health care adopted FMEA in the late 1990s.

Definitions for HFMEA include:

1. *HFMEA:* Healthcare Failure Mode and Effects Analysis.

2. *Failure mode:* The way in which each identified failure occurs (e.g., wrong medication administered to the patient, wrong dosage of medication administered to the patient, wrong route of drug administered to the patient).

3. *Effects:* The final result (outcome/effect) that may occur from the failure mode (e.g., Adverse or Sentinel Event).

4. *(S) Severity Score:* A score that is assigned for the worst-case scenario of what can happen when the failure mode occurs. The higher the severity score, the more likely the effects will cause harm to the patient.

5. *(O) Occurrence (probability):* How many times the failure mode is likely to occur. A higher number means that the chance of recurrence is higher.

6. *(D) Detection:* How likely the failure is to be detected before it reaches the patient. A high detection number means that the chances are high that the failure will escape detection.

7. *RPN:* After numbers are assigned for severity, occurrence, and detectability; the RPN is calculated. This score is obtained by multiplying: $RPN = S \times O \times D$. High RPNs need efforts to obtain the best

TABLE 14.2
Comparison of FMEA to RCA

	FMEA	RCA
Process	X	
Case study		X
Prospective	X	
Retrospective		X

possible solutions with error-proofing methods as recommended actions.

FMEA looks at what can go wrong, how likely it is to go wrong, and what the consequences are when it does go wrong.

The consequences are the probability that the scenario will yield the worst possible consequences. Risk is calculated by multiplying the severity with the probability.

The FMEA approach maps out the process and the subprocesses. For each step, an analysis is completed. The analysis covers the ways in which the process/subprocesses may fail or the manner in which the failure may occur (failure modes).

The Joint Commission requires at least one proactive risk assessment on an annual basis for an identified high-risk process.

The basic steps for HFMEA are:

1. Select and define the high-risk clinical process in which HFMEA will be used.
2. Form a multidisciplinary team who have knowledge of the process, and have an expert facilitator provide just-in-time training if needed, prior to starting the HFMEA process.
3. Map out the current process and subprocesses.
4. Identify the failure modes and assign severity, occurrence probability, and detectability scores.
5. Assign RPNs by multiplying the severity, occurrence, and detectability scores.
6. Develop risk reduction methods using error-proofing methods and redesign the process to prevent failures or to intercept adverse events.
7. Test the new process.
8. Implement and monitor the redesigned process (develop effective outcome measures).

There are variations in the process for performing HFMEA; however, the principles remain constant.

The VA has the most widely disseminated tools for conducting HFMEA. The VA combined the U.S. FDA's Hazard Analysis and Critical Point (HACCP) tool together with components from the VA's RCA process. The free forms to use for each step of the process are available at www.patientsafety.gov/safetytopics.html.

The IHI has a lot of information, including case studies for implementing HFMEAs at http://www.ihi.org/Pages/default.aspx. Search FMEA.

The ISMP has sample HFMEAs; the one for anticoagulants is available at www.ismp.org/Tools/anticoagulantTherapy.asp.

In 2002, the ASHRM produced a white paper titled "Strategies and Tips for Maximizing Failure Mode and Effects Analysis in Your Organization," which you will find in Appendix B. It contains tips for risk managers along with the steps for HFMEA.

CONCLUSION

RCA provides a detailed analysis of why the adverse event occurred. There is a systematic process for conducting a credible and thorough RCA. The focus is on the system, not on the individual. Cases of reckless behavior are handled through administrative channels. Aggregation of root cause cases is strongly recommended to enable clarification of patterns and an enhanced search for further opportunities for risk reduction.

FMEA is a proactive, prospective method to analyze the vulnerabilities in a process and control or eliminate them. FMEA is a tool that assists to increase reliability of processes. The Joint Commission requires only one FMEA every 18 months.

REFERENCES

Agency for Healthcare Research and Quality . (n.d.). *Patient safety primer: Root cause analysis.* Retrieved June 28, 2010, from http://www.psnet.ahrq.gov/primer.aspx?primerID=10

Canadian Patient Safety Institute. (2006). *Canadian root cause analysis framework: A tool for identifying and addressing the root causes of critical incidents in healthcare.* Retrieved June 28, 2010, from http://www.patientsafety institute.ca/English/toolsresources/rca/Documents/March%20 2006%20RCA%20Workbook.pdf

Joint Commission. (2009). *Sentinel event policy and procedures; Updated 2007.* Retrieved June 28, 2010, from http://www.jointcommission.org/ Sentinel_Event_Policy_and_Procedures/

National Center for Patient Safety. (n.d.). *Glossary of patient safety terms.* Retrieved June 28, 2010, from http://www.patientsafety.gov/glossary.html

Stalhandske, E., De Rosier, J., Wilson, R., & Murphy, J. (2009). *Healthcare FMEA in the veterans health administration.* Retrieved 27 June, 2010, from http://www.psqh.com/septemberoctober-2009/239-healthcare-fmea-in-the-veterans-health-administration.html

V

Recommendations for Future Consideration

15

Recommendations for Accrediting Bodies and Health Care Organizations

*A*ccrediting bodies are proliferating internationally for many reasons. Medical tourism is one driver; patients going overseas to obtain cheaper health care than what is offered in the United States is another driver.

In 2008, Erbeck, Guevara, and Mango reported that the current market for medical tourism is between 60,000 and 85,000 inpatients per year. Comparisons of cost are significant. An aortic valve replacement, for example, which costs more than $100,000 in the United States, compares to only $12,000 at a provider in Asia. And while the largest, current barrier to medical tourism is the insurer's reluctance to include overseas health care organizations within their networks, other barriers also exist, including the lack of performance measures for outcomes and issues surrounding various patient rights when adverse outcomes occur within each country.

The world is becoming increasingly complex and the future may hold an international perspective and market for health care accreditation and patient safety. In this regard, it is significant to recall that the ISQua, the only global body that accredits the accreditors of health care, initiated its international accreditation program in 1999.

As of March 2010, ISQua has accredited 17 organizations along with 31 sets of standards from 23 organizations. The accreditation of five surveyor training programs has also been included here. Fortunately, ISQua's standards, *International Standards for Healthcare External Evaluation Organisations*, provide a generic systems framework that accrediting bodies use to develop their own specific health care standards.

The Joint Commission received ISQua accreditation in September 2000. The Joint Commission is the leader in international hospital accreditation since 1994 (Joint Commission, n.d.).

According to WHO (2004), health systems operate within an environment "of rapid social, economic and technological change. Such changes are expected to continue for the foreseeable future as a result of restructured economic and social policies, globalization of markets and enhanced communication. Many health systems currently in place have neglected evaluation of the quality of individual and systematic institutional care in the past, giving rise to an unnecessary increase in costs. Accreditation can be the single most important approach for improving the quality of health care structures."

To continue to drive patient safety efforts and make health care safer, there needs to be a systems approach.

From the evidence presented within the Myers Model for Patient Safety and Accreditation, six key recommendations for all accrediting bodies arise:

1. There needs to be consideration for creating new standards that measure an engaged workforce; this will require assessments related to the quality of worklife for employees.

   An engaged workforce is essential for transforming health care into a high-reliability organization. Health care organizations need to ensure that caring is integrated into the work, for patients and for staff.

2. There needs to be consideration for higher accountability at the leadership level. Standards related to evidence of teamwork at the leadership level must be developed. Also, standards to evaluate the leadership's involvement in role-modeling values that demonstrate congruence in building patient safety cultures would greatly enhance safety efforts.

3. There needs to be greater encouragement and sharing of RPI methods with centralized areas for sharing of information. The Joint Commission's Center for Transforming Healthcare shares information on their RPI projects with participating hospitals. To see the latest information, go to http://www.centerfortransforminghealthcare.org/methodologies/default.aspx

4. There need to be standards that measure if a safe environment is present for employees (e.g., restrictions for mandatory overtime, interventions that prevent preventable employee injuries).
5. There need to be educational requirements for the leadership that include their knowledge regarding patient safety concepts and RPI.
6. There needs to be consideration of an annual award to the top 10 hospitals or health care systems that have the best quality of worklife as measured by an independent survey.

Accrediting bodies have the opportunity to share information on quality and patient safety improvement efforts with each other using ISQua as a forum to compare the unique features of each accrediting body.

The Myers Model for Patient Safety and Accreditation can be used by accrediting bodies as they strive to move their patient safety agenda forward. This is accomplished by raising the bar of expected performance through application of standards. The information can be used at consensus workshops and other forums with stakeholders to revise and/or develop new standards.

RECOMMENDATIONS FOR HEALTH CARE ORGANIZATIONS

Hospitals in the United States have been merging and growing for many years. According to Yonek, Hines, and Joshi (2010), multi-hospital health care systems are the most common organizational structures in the United States. There are 200 hospital systems (defined as having two or more general acute care hospitals) that comprise half of all hospitals and hospital admissions in the United States.

Dissatisfaction of health care workers is on the rise, and past downsizing initiatives have led to a general mistrust in the environment. Staff may be reluctant to fully participate in quality and patient safety efforts due to fear of job insecurity.

Employees may also wonder why the environment cannot be made safer for them. For example, according to the *American Journal of Critical Care*, approximately 9,000 health care workers sustain a disabling injury every day. The primary root cause of these injuries is lifting patients (Brown, 2003).

Workplace violence in higher-risk areas, such as emergency rooms, needs a higher priority for interventions. It is not acceptable to have health care professionals experiencing preventable injuries in the workplace.

Hospital leadership has an ethical obligation to ensure safety within the workplace. If workers are not safe, then how can we hope that our patients will be safe?

Leaders are trusted to do the right thing. When employees lose trust in leadership, the work environment becomes toxic. Employees wonder why they don't get pay raises and yet they see more hospital expansions taking place. When employees are not treated as valuable human capital, employee engagement will be low. If employees perform only up to minimal compliance, it will not be conducive to having a highly performing workforce.

As a remedy, the Myers Model for Patient Safety and Accreditation provides nine recommendations for health care institutions:

1. Make employee satisfaction a priority. Assess the quality of worklife and improve it.
2. Consider innovative leader models such as joint leadership or team leadership, where power is shared.
3. Provide the necessary resources at the unit level to drive accountability and pay particular attention to information systems that have the capability to provide the team current information on quality and patient safety metrics.
4. Ensure that the leadership is visible and works as an effective team. Health care is too complex to work alone.
5. Make employee safety a priority (both physical and psychological). There should be zero preventable employee injuries/deaths.
6. Use the Myers Model for Patient Safety and Accreditation current evidence on each element in the system and assess if implementation is warranted.
7. Develop a set of outcome measurements as identified in the Myers Model for Patient Safety and Accreditation to gauge if your organization's patient safety interventions are effective.
8. Determine which accrediting body will provide the most value to drive patient safety efforts within your organization.
9. Ensure that your nurse executive and the rest of the leadership team stay longer than 2 to 3 years. It takes time to build relationships and form a high-performing team. This executive group is critical to ongoing success.

CONCLUSION

The quality of worklife for employees must improve in order to develop and maintain a satisfied and engaged work force.

To achieve this, leaders should use a systems-based approach instead of solving one problem at a time with isolated views. Incremental change is simply not enough—hospital leaders need to take big steps forward now; the patient safety model will assist them to make the right decisions.

It takes a committed, engaged workforce to transform health care into what it should have been all along—safe, effective, timely, efficient, equitable, and patient centered.

Dr. Berwick stated, "Some is not a number; soon is not a time." Where patient safety is concerned, *Zero is the number*—no adverse events for patients or staff.

Today, health care leaders need to revisit their strategic plans using the Myers Model for Patient Safety and Accreditation as a guide. Accrediting bodies need to use the model for raising the bar for expectations of performance related to patient safety.

More than 10 years since the IOM's first shocking report on medical errors was published, *NOW is the time*— NOW is today.

REFERENCES

American Nurses Association's (2010). *Mandatory overtime.* Retrieved August 10, 2010, from http://www.nursingworld.org/MainMenuCategories/ANAPoliticalPower/State/StateLegislativeAgenda/MandatoryOvertime.aspx.

Berwick, D. M. (2005). *Some is not a number: Soon is not a time.* AHQA Annual Meeting and Technical Conference. San Franciso: Institute for Healthcare Improvement.

Brown, D. (2003). Nurses and preventable back injuries. *American Journal of Critical Care.* Retrieved August 10, 2010, from http://ajcc.aacnjournals.org/cgi/content/full/12/5/400

Erbeck, T., Guevara, C., & Mango, P. D. (2008). *Mapping the market for medical travel. Health care.* Retrieved August 12, 2010, from http://www.health-tourism.com/medical-tourism/statistics/.

International Society for Quality in Health Care (2010). Accreditation. *What is ISQua's international accreditation proramme?* Retrieved August 12, 2010, from http://www.isqua.org/accreditations.htm.

Joint Commission. (n.d.) *About joint commission international.* Retrieved August 12, 2010, from http://www.jointcommissioninternational.org/About-JCI/.

WHO Regional Office for the Eastern Mediterranean. (2004). *Hospital accreditation.* Retrieved August 12, 2010, from http://www.emro.who.int/mei/HA.htm.

Yonek, J., Hines, S., & Joshi, M. A. (2010). *A guide to achieving high performance in multi-hospital health systems.* Health Research & Educational Trust. Retrieved August 2, 2010, from http://www.aha.org/aha/resource-center/Statistics-and-Studies/studies.html.

Appendix A

Safe Practices for Better Healthcare—2010 Update: A Consensus Report

EXECUTIVE SUMMARY

Now a decade after the Institute of Medicine's report *To Err is Human*, some advances have been made in patient safety, yet the consensus is clear that there is still much to do. With the recognition that healthcare-associated infections are for the most part preventable, and that zero infections is the number we must chase, medical-related harm as the leading cause of death in America has not gone down, but gone up from the eighth leading cause in 1999 to the third leading cause.

The Safe Practices for Better Healthcare – 2010 Update presents 34 practices that have been demonstrated to be effective in reducing the occurrence of adverse healthcare events. The practices are organized into seven functional categories for improving patient safety:

- creating and sustaining a culture of safety (Chapter 2);
- informed consent, life-sustaining treatment, disclosure, and care of the caregiver (Chapter 3);
- matching healthcare needs with service delivery capability (Chapter 4);

- facilitating information transfer and clear communication (Chapter 5);
- medication management (Chapter 6);
- prevention of healthcare-associated infections (Chapter 7); and
- condition- and site-specific practices (Chapter 8).

Based on feedback from healthcare organizations, subject matter experts, and the NQF Safe Practices Consensus Committee, the 2010 update has made modest changes to the 2009 report.

In Chapters 2 through 8, the problem statements, implementation approach information, and other narrative elements that do not constitute the endorsed standards have been significantly updated. No substantive changes were made to the latest additional specifications. Chapter 9 describes selected contributions from patient advocate experts as examples of the themes that are believed to be important for patients and families to consider during their healthcare encounters. Specific recommendations regarding patients and families are embodied formally in each practice. This section has been modestly updated with input from patient advocates and organizations that have embraced the concept of involving patients and families in their safety and quality programs.

As with the previously endorsed practices, these 34 safe practices should be universally utilized in applicable healthcare settings to reduce the risk of harm resulting from processes, systems, and environments of care.

This set of safe practices is not intended to capture all activities that might reduce adverse healthcare events. Rather, this report continues the focus on practices that:

- have strong evidence that they are effective in reducing the likelihood of harming a patient;
- are generalizable (i.e., they may be applied in multiple clinical care settings and/or for multiple types of patients);
- are likely to have a significant benefit to patient safety if fully implemented; and
- have knowledge about them that consumers, purchasers, providers, and researchers can use.

The implementation of these practices will improve patient safety. Additionally, other important uses of the set are to help healthcare providers assess the degree to which safe practices already have been implemented in their settings and to assess the degree to which the practices provide tangible evidence of patient safety improvement and increased patient satisfaction and loyalty. And importantly, with this update, healthcare organization leaders and governance boards are explicitly called upon to proactively review the safety of their organizations and to take action to improve continually the safety and thus the quality of care they provide.

The safe practices are not prioritized or weighted within or across categories. This is because all are viewed as important in improving patient safety and because no objective, evidence-based method of prioritizing the practices could be identified that would equitably apply across the current heterogeneous universe of healthcare organizations that have variably implemented many—and in some cases all—of these practices. For any given healthcare provider, the choice of priority practices for implementation will depend on the provider's circumstances, including which of the practices already have been implemented, the degree of success the provider has had with implementation, the availability of resources, environmental constraints, and other factors.

This report does not represent the entire scope of NQF work pertinent to improving patient safety and healthcare quality; over the years since the publication of the original set of safe practices, NQF has completed and updated a number of projects of direct relevance to this report. In 2006, NQF endorsed 28 serious reportable events in healthcare that should be reported by all licensed healthcare facilities. In 2007, NQF completed a consensus project related to the assessment and prevention of healthcare-associated infections (HAIs). The HAI report specifically called for additional practices in HAI prevention, with a specific call for a new safe practice related to catheter-associated urinary tract infections. NQF also endorsed a set of Patient Safety Indicators developed by the Agency for Healthcare Research and Quality. Additional safety-related work included focused projects on perioperative care, the prevention of venous thromboembolism, a pressure ulcer prevention framework, and the endorsement of measures related to patient safety and medication management. Finally, the emerging priorities and goals from the National Priorities Partnership include a strong focus on avoidable harm, continuity of care, and patient safety.

TABLE A.1
Safe Practices for Better Healthcare-2010 Update

SAFE PRACTICE	PRACTICE STATEMENT
Safe Practice 1: Leadership Structures and Systems	Leadership structures and systems must be established to ensure that there is organization-wide awareness of patient safety performance gaps, direct accountability of leaders for those gaps, and adequate investment in performance improvement abilities, and that actions are taken to ensure safe care of every patient served.
Safe Practice 2: Culture Measurement, Feedback, and Intervention	Healthcare organizations must measure their culture, provide feedback to the leadership and staff, and undertake interventions that will reduce patient safety risk.
Safe Practice 3: Teamwork Training and Skill Building	Healthcare organizations must establish a proactive, systematic, organization-wide approach to developing team-based care through teamwork training, skill building, and team-led performance improvement interventions that reduce preventable harm to patients.
Safe Practice 4: Identification and Mitigation of Risks and Hazards	Healthcare organizations must systematically identify and mitigate patient safety risks and hazards with an integrated approach in order to continuously drive down preventable patient harm.
Safe Practice 5: Informed Consent	Ask each patient or legal surrogate to "teach back," in his or her own words, key information about the proposed treatments or procedures for which he or she is being asked to provide informed consent.
Safe Practice 6: Life-Sustaining Treatment	Ensure that written documentation of the patient's preferences for life-sustaining treatments is prominently displayed in his or her chart.
Safe Practice 7: Disclosure	Following serious unanticipated outcomes, including those that are clearly caused by systems failures, the patient and, as appropriate, the family should receive timely, transparent, and clear communication concerning what is known about the event.
Safe Practice 8: Care of the Caregiver	Following serious unintentional harm due to systems failures and/or errors that resulted from human performance failures, the involved caregivers (clinical providers, staff, and administrators) should receive timely and systematic care to include: treatment that is just, respect, compassion, supportive medical care, and the opportunity to fully participate in event investigation and risk identification and mitigation activities that will prevent future events.

SAFE PRACTICE	PRACTICE STATEMENT
Safe Practice 9: Nursing Workforce	Implement critical components of a well-designed nursing workforce that mutually reinforce patient safeguards, including the following: ■ A nurse staffing plan with evidence that it is adequately resourced and actively managed and that its effectiveness is regularly evaluated with respect to patient safety. ■ Senior administrative nursing leaders, such as a Chief Nursing Officer, as part of the hospital senior management team. ■ Governance boards and senior administrative leaders that take accountability for reducing patient safety risks related to nurse staffing decisions and the provision of financial resources for nursing services. ■ Provision of budgetary resources to support nursing staff in the ongoing acquisition and maintenance of professional knowledge and skills.
Safe Practice 10: Direct Caregivers	Ensure that non-nursing direct care staffing levels are adequate, that the staff are competent, and that they have had adequate orientation, training, and education to perform their assigned direct care duties.
Safe Practice 11: Intensive Care Unit Care	All patients in general intensive care units (both adult and pediatric) should be managed by physicians who have specific training and certification in critical care medicine ("critical care certified").
Safe Practice 12: Patient Care Information	Ensure that care information is transmitted and appropriately documented in a timely manner and in a clearly understandable form to patients and to all of the patient's healthcare providers/ professionals, within and between care settings, who need that information to provide continued care.
Safe Practice 13: Order Read-Back and Abbreviations	Incorporate within your organization a safe, effective communication strategy, structures, and systems to include the following: ■ For verbal or telephone orders or for telephonic reporting of critical test results, verify the complete order or test result by having the person who is receiving the information record and "read-back" the complete order or test result. ■ Standardize a list of "Do Not Use" abbreviations, acronyms, symbols, and dose designations that cannot be used throughout the organization.

(continued)

TABLE A.1 (*continued*)

SAFE PRACTICE	PRACTICE STATEMENT
Safe Practice 14: Labeling of Diagnostic Studies	Implement standardized policies, processes, and systems to ensure accurate labeling of radiographs, laboratory specimens, or other diagnostic studies, so that the right study is labeled for the right patient at the right time.
Safe Practice 15: Discharge Systems	A "discharge plan" must be prepared for each patient at the time of hospital discharge, and a concise discharge summary must be prepared for and relayed to the clinical caregiver accepting responsibility for postdischarge care in a timely manner. Organizations must ensure that there is confirmation of receipt of the discharge information by the independent licensed practitioner who will assume the responsibility for care after discharge.
Safe Practice 16: Safe Adoption of Computerized Prescriber Order Entry	Implement a computerized prescriber order entry (CPOE) system built upon the requisite foundation of re-engineered evidence-based care, an assurance of healthcare organization staff and independent practitioner readiness, and an integrated information technology infrastructure.
Safe Practice 17: Medication Reconciliation	The healthcare organization must develop, reconcile, and communicate an accurate patient medication list throughout the continuum of care.
Safe Practice 18: Pharmacist Leadership Structures and Systems	Pharmacy leaders should have an active role on the administrative leadership team that reflects their authority and accountability for medication management systems performance across the organization.
Safe Practice 19: Hand Hygiene	Comply with current Centers for Disease Control and Prevention Hand Hygiene Guidelines.
Safe Practice 20: Influenza Prevention	Comply with current Centers for Disease Control and Prevention (CDC) recommendations for influenza vaccinations for healthcare personnel and the annual recommendations of the CDC Advisory Committee on Immunization Practices for individual influenza prevention and control.
Safe Practice 21: Central Line-Associated Bloodstream Infection Prevention	Take actions to prevent central line-associated bloodstream infection by implementing evidence-based intervention practices.
Safe Practice 22: Surgical-Site Infection Prevention	Take actions to prevent surgical-site infections by implementing evidence-based intervention practices. Safe Practice 22 is currently under ad hoc review by an expert panel. This practice will be updated in the coming months to reflect the review decision.

SAFE PRACTICE	PRACTICE STATEMENT
Safe Practice 23: Care of the Ventilated Patient	Take actions to prevent complications associated with ventilated patients: specifically, ventilator-associated pneumonia, venous thromboembolism, peptic ulcer disease, dental complications, and pressure ulcers.
Safe Practice 24: Multidrug-Resistant Organism Prevention	Implement a systematic multidrug-resistant organism (MDRO) eradication program built upon the fundamental elements of infection control, an evidence-based approach, assurance of the hospital staff and independent practitioner readiness, and a re-engineered identification and care process for those patients with or at risk for MDRO infections. Note: This practice applies to, but is not limited to, epidemiologically important organisms such as methicillin-resistant Staphylococcus aureus, vancomycin-resistant enterococci, and Clostridium difficile. Multidrug-resistant gram-negative bacilli, such as Enterobacter species, Klebsiella species, Pseudomonas species, and Escherichia coli, and vancomycin-resistant Staphylococcus aureus, should be evaluated for inclusion on a local system level based on organizational risk assessments.
Safe Practice 25: Catheter-Associated Urinary Tract Infection Prevention	Take actions to prevent catheter-associated urinary tract infection by implementing evidence-based intervention practices.
Safe Practice 26: Wrong-Site, Wrong-Procedure, Wrong-Person Surgery Prevention	Implement the Universal Protocol for Preventing Wrong Site, Wrong Procedure, Wrong Person Surgery™ for all invasive procedures.
Safe Practice 27: Pressure Ulcer Prevention	Take actions to prevent pressure ulcers by implementing evidence-based intervention practices.
Safe Practice 28: Venous Thromboembolism Prevention	Evaluate each patient upon admission, and regularly thereafter, for the risk of developing venous thromboembolism. Utilize clinically appropriate, evidence-based methods of thromboprophylaxis.
Safe Practice 29: Anticoagulation Therapy	Organizations should implement practices to prevent patient harm due to anticoagulant therapy.
Safe Practice 30: Contrast Media-Induced Renal Failure Prevention	Utilize validated protocols to evaluate patients who are at risk for contrast media-induced renal failure and gadolinium-associated nephrogenic systemic fibrosis, and utilize a clinically appropriate method for reducing the risk of adverse events based on the patient's risk evaluations.

(continued)

TABLE A.1 (*continued*)

SAFE PRACTICE	PRACTICE STATEMENT
Safe Practice 31: Organ Donation	Hospital policies that are consistent with applicable law and regulations should be in place and should address patient and family preferences for organ donation, as well as specify the roles and desired outcomes for every stage of the donation process.
Safe Practice 32: Glycemic Control	Take actions to improve glycemic control by implementing evidence-based intervention practices that prevent hypoglycemia and optimize the care of patients with hyperglycemia and diabetes.
Safe Practice 33: Falls Prevention	Take actions to prevent patient falls and to reduce fall-related injuries by implementing evidence-based intervention practices.
Safe Practice 34: Pediatric Imaging	When CT imaging studies are undertaken on children, "child-size" techniques should be used to reduce unnecessary exposure to ionizing radiation.

Appendix B

Strategies and Tips for Maximizing Failure Mode & Effect Analysis in Your Organization

*T*he prevention and reduction of errors in the provision of healthcare have captured the increased attention of policymakers, providers, and the public over the past ten years. As research into patient safety has become more sophisticated and the healthcare community has embraced fields of study outside of healthcare, a shift in thinking about how errors occur has provided new ways to approach possible solutions.

Patient safety is, arguably, a traditional risk management concept viewed in a contemporary format. One definition of healthcare is about loss control, whether human loss or financial loss, and has been at the foundation of every successful risk management program since the inception of risk management. Risk assessment and risk treatment tools used by risk managers have evolved over time and include both reactive and proactive measures. As new thinking, strategies, tools, and practices have been launched, risk managers have eagerly accepted these changes in their commitment to reducing risk in healthcare organizations.

For example, there are various techniques used in industry and aerospace for conducting proactive risk assessment. These risk assessment techniques have recently become recognized for their relevance

Printed with permission from *American Society for Healthcare Risk Management.*

to healthcare. The most widely known tool that incorporates methods for identifying failure modes and their causes is one developed and used in the aerospace industry since the mid-1960's—Failure Mode and Effect Analysis (FMEA).[1]

Applied to healthcare, FMEA is one patient safety tool that provides risk managers the opportunity to "get ahead of the curve" and favorably impact the patient care environment. The Joint Commission on Accreditation of Healthcare Organizations (JCAHO) is a leading driver behind the use of FMEA. In 2001, the JCAHO revised its accreditation standards to include a requirement that healthcare organizations perform, annually, at least one proactive risk assessment on a high-risk process. While the standard, LD 5.2[2], does not mandate that a specific proactive risk assessment methodology be used, such as FMEA, it does outline a generic process for identifying and addressing failure modes in healthcare processes.

INTRODUCING FMEA

This paper will refer to FMEA and HFMEA™ (Healthcare Failure Mode Effect Analysis) interchangeably. HFMEA™ refers to the terminology developed specifically for use in healthcare by the Veterans Administration National Center for Patient Safety (VA NCPS) with assistance from the Tenet Health System. The paper will not teach you how to conduct an FMEA or HFMEA™ but instead will take you through the steps of risk assessment and provide a framework for understanding.

This paper will describe how to use proactive risk assessment for patient safety, when to use it, and who should be involved in its application. It will also explore concerns about evidentiary protection and discoverability. Lastly, this paper will provide risk management tips from risk managers in the field who are facilitating failure mode analyses.

The VA NCPS extensively reviewed several proactive risk assessment tools before determining that the application of such tools in healthcare required some modification. As such, the VA NCPS has modified the concepts of FMEA and deployed the techniques and tools in all of its 163 healthcare centers. The new tool was named HFMEA™.

---

[1]The Basics of FMEA; R. McDermott, R. Mikulak, M. Beauregard; 1996; p. 3
[2]JCAHO 2002 Hospital Accreditation Standard, LD 5.2, p. 200–201

The American Hospital Association has recently mailed a package of HFMEA™ materials to every hospital CEO in the country. The package includes video and CD instruction and worksheets on the use and application of HFMEA™. The materials in the kit are intended to be shared with risk managers and others in the organization responsible for patient safety.

Traditionally, failure mode refers to a weakness or vulnerability in any part of a process or a chain of events that has the potential to cause a safety problem. Failure occurs when a process begins to produce something you don't want. HFMEA™ looks at a process, as is typically done in healthcare where FMEA, traditionally used in industry to assist in the recognition and identification of potential failure modes, looks at a device or component. In either application, the use allows for a proactive examination of what could go wrong and the opportunity to fix it before failure. As used in healthcare, both are adaptations of previously prescribed methodologies that, while used predominantly in certain fields in the past, are not specific to any particular application. Both FMEA and HFMEA™ can be used to meet the intent of the JCAHO standard for proactive risk assessment. They are consistent with, but not necessarily inclusive of, the requirements of the standard.

WHAT DOES FMEA MEAN FOR RISK MANAGERS?

Risk managers are experienced and knowledgeable about investigating medical errors and developing strategies and deploying tools to improve patient safety. FMEA is another tool in the box of effective risk management strategies to understand and reduce medical errors. Where the advent of sentinel event reporting and performing of root cause analysis bolsters the tenet of "learning from our mistakes," FMEA assists risk managers and others in driving change before it can do harm by forecasting potential failures and proactively applying loss control techniques to those potential failures. To do this, risk managers and others in an organization must conduct an in-depth analysis of a process in order to assess and modify it to reduce the potential for harm.

FMEA—GETTING STARTED

What follows is an overview of one particular method of proactive risk assessment—FMEA.

Select a High-Risk Process

Strategy
Develop a list of high-risk processes in your organization. From the list, select one or more processes (or sub-processes) for which to perform an FMEA. Processes that have variable input, are complex, non-standardized, heavily dependent on human intervention, performed under tight or loose time constraints, tightly coupled and hierarchical (not team oriented) are all candidates for consideration.

Risk Management Tips:

- In identifying processes for proactive risk assessment, consider incident reports, loss experience/claims data, worker's compensation reports, the literature, or anything that even intuitively, warrants analysis. Consider, also, those accidents that have high severity or occur with great frequency. Catastrophic events are sentinel events and any of the Sentinel Event Alerts issued by the JCAHO may yield opportunities for possible analysis.
- Keep a "parking lot" list of your ideas for possible analysis.
- While the JCAHO standard requires that at least one proactive risk assessment be performed each year, your organization may benefit from conducting as many as possible given limits on organizational resources.
- Be realistic about the scope of the high-risk process or sub-process you identify for risk assessment – start small so that you and your team are not overwhelmed. Don't look for problems that don't exist.
- Get support from senior leadership.

Assemble a Team

Strategy
The team should consist of a multidisciplinary group of people, including physicians, who regularly perform the activity identified as high-risk. While the size of the team can vary depending on the number of people involved in a process, be prudent by including those with hands-on experience, and keep the team small. Other important members of the team include a subject matter expert, a leader, and a facilitator who understands the FMEA process. It is also important to include a neutral party — a person who is not intimately familiar with

the process but whose perspective will be helpful to thinking outside of the box.

Risk Management Tips:

- The role of the risk manager may be multifaceted. The risk manager may be the leader, the facilitator or the content expert. It is advisable, though, that the risk manager avoids being the leader and the facilitator concurrently in order to manage the workload.
- A subject matter expert is a person who owns or plays a major role in the process chosen for assessment.
- A leader is a person who has experience with guiding a team and who will lead the team to ensure risk reduction is completed.
- A facilitator is a person who is trained to understand team dynamics, is knowledgeable about the FMEA process, and can advise the leader throughout the assessment. A good facilitator is important to open communication.
- It is important for team members to know what they will gain from the experience. Involve them in developing a schedule and give them ownership.
- There are many good resources to learn more about creating high performing teams. One to consider is *The Team Handbook* by Scholtes, Joiner, and Striebel.

Diagram the Process

Strategy
Once the team has agreed upon the process to examine, map the process by using flowcharting or cause and effect diagramming techniques that are understood in the organization. Identify the "way things were intended to work" and the "way things are actually working."

Risk Management Tips:

- Do your homework — conduct literature searches on the topic for risk assessment. Identify best practices, review/refer to internal procedures and policies, and look outside your organization for information.

(continued)

(continued)

■ There are many good resources to learn more about flowcharting, cause and effect diagramming and other mapping techniques. One to consider is *The Memory Jogger* by Brassard and Ritter.

■ Use Post-it™ notes or self-adhesive index cards to track the steps. Use a wall or whiteboard to post the notes (representing the steps in the process) to create a visual representation of the process being assessed.

■ Invite the team to visit the worksite and observe the process.

Identify the Potential Failure Modes

Strategy

Identify the steps in the process where there is, or may be, undesirable variation. The gap between the ideal and the reality are often the first failure modes identified. A process can have multiple failure modes and each failure mode can have multiple possible effects. In reviewing each step in the process, the following questions should be addressed:

1. What could fail with this step? (i.e., failure modes)
2. Why would this failure occur? (i.e., causes)
3. What could happen if this failure occurred? (i.e., effects)

Risk Management Tips:

■ Code (number, letter, color) each step in the process. Include sub-processes.

■ Allowing for ample team discussion is an effective way for the team to identify failure modes. As a quality improvement tool, brainstorming has certain rules that should be followed to maximize its effectiveness and assure full participation by all.

Assess Failure Modes and Identify Causes

Strategy

Fundamental risk assessment is grounded in identification and measurement of risk. Measuring, or ranking, risk is facilitated by using a pre-determined methodology that is understood and consistently applied in an organization. To mitigate risk, you must understand the frequency and severity of that risk.

HFMEA™ uses a simplified tool, the Hazard Scoring Matrix™, to assess risk. The Matrix applies hazard analysis principles that factor in the severity and probability of the potential failure mode occurring. The severity score is a "measure of the potential effect of the failure mode." The Matrix defines degrees of severity as: catastrophic, major, moderate, and minor. Degrees of probability are defined as frequent, occasional, uncommon, and remote.[3]

In the industry model of FMEA, each failure is assigned a risk priority number (RPN) based on the likelihood of occurrence (OC), the severity if it occurred (SV), and the likelihood of detection (DT). RPN = OC x SV x DT.

When ranking risk, other factors can be considered. The JCAHO is not specific as to how to prioritize the failure modes for further analysis and action, but expects some sort of ranking so that limited resources will be applied in the most useful manner.

Risk Management Tips:

- Keep track of definitions that are used for rating risk and use them consistently.
- Use a common nomenclature when describing, discussing, and applying the rating tool.
- Consider a catastrophic event to be nearly the same as a sentinel event. Keep the scale simple.

Conduct a Root Cause Analysis (RCA) on
the Most Critical Failure Modes

Strategy
Failures with the highest score are those that should be focused on first. The team should look at the potential root causes of the highly scored failure by asking the following questions:

1. Why might the failure occur?

2. When might the failure occur?

---

[3]JCAHO *Journal on Quality Improvement;* May 2002 Journal, Volume 28, Number 5; page 254.

3. What might cause the failure to occur? (i.e., steps in the process)

4. Where might the failure occur?

It is important to note the differences between root cause analysis and FMEA/HFMEA™. Both have the goal to reduce patient harm, involve identifying conditions that lead to harm, and are team activities. However, they are distinct in that FMEA/HFMEA™ is proactive, focuses on an entire process and asks "what if?" The root cause analysis is reactive, focuses on the actual failure, is clarified by hindsight, prone to fear and resistance, and asks "why?" It may be helpful to use RCA as part of the FMEA process when it is necessary to analyze failure modes that do not have immediately evident actionable causes. To reduce risk, it's important to understand the root causes of the failure

Redesign the Process

Strategy

Use mapping techniques such as flowcharts, fishbone, and cause and effect diagrams and as much discussion as needed to identify and design the new process. Actions for the team to consider in the redesign of the process include:

1. Determine if a step in the process should be eliminated, controlled, transferred, or accepted.

2. Identify an action or countermeasure for the failure mode that would reduce future risk

3. Choose a person to complete the action.

4. Identify the process or approach to reduce the risk.

Risk Management Tips:

- As the process is redesigned, apply principles of patient safety such as reducing reliance on memory; incorporating the use of checklists and protocols; incorporating redundancy; improving information access; reducing hand-offs; standardizing procedures, displays and layouts; using forcing functions, and simplifying procedures.
- Take a break then come back to perform another FMEA on the redesigned process before widespread implementation.

- Conduct a literature review to identify any recommended risk reduction strategies that have already been successfully implemented.
- Pilot test the redesigned process before widespread implementation.

Identify and implement Measures of Effectiveness

Strategy
After the new process is implemented and staff is trained in the new process, the new process needs to be measured to see if it is improved.

Risk Management Tips:

- Conduct audits. Interviewing or reconvening members of the team performing the new process is critical to measure effectiveness.
- Provide feedback to the team. Doing so can be an effective incentive for team members to continue to participate in proactive risk assessment.
- Observe the new process and map it to compare it to the ideal.
- Employ project management software.
- Depending on the risk manager's responsibilities, decide if the ongoing monitoring of the new process may be more appropriately handled by PI personnel so quality indicators can be used to measure improvement.

Implement a Strategy of Maintaining the Effectiveness of the Redesigned Process Over Time.

Strategy
Measure the process again.

Risk Management Tips:

- Periodically check in with team members.

Protecting the Process

As with root cause analysis, the potential use of an FMEA generated document by a plaintiff in a legal action alleging medical malpractice is of great concern to many risk managers. The concern is, perhaps, heightened because FMEA proactively identifies potential failures and assigns a hazard score or risk priority number. To the extent that identified potential failures are not addressed (or not addressed well) and there is a later mishap involving that particular failure point, a previously existing FMEA could provide potent evidence for a plaintiff in a medical malpractice case (provided that the FMEA is subject to discovery and is admissible in court). Obviously, such a result would have a chilling effect on an organization's future use of FMEA for proactive risk assessment.

Risk managers can mitigate the potential discovery of FMEA and other sources of organizational analysis by following procedures under state laws that permit limited discovery protections for work product related to peer review or quality improvement. Under most states' law, these peer review or quality improvement protections are provided to promote the important public policy that furthers organizational self-evaluation of medical errors and systems improvement. In addition, some organizations perform FMEA at the direction of legal counsel, thereby creating attorney-client privilege.

Although some states provide limited protection for work products related to peer review or quality improvement, this protection under the patchwork of state laws is subject to judicial interpretation and balancing of a plaintiff's interest in discovery versus the public policy interest promoted by the peer review or quality improvement statute.

Currently, there are limited federal statutes promoting the public policy interests that further peer review and quality improvement activities in healthcare organizations. However, the Patient Safety and Quality Improvement Act (S. 2590), recently introduced in the Senate, seeks legal protections for information submitted voluntarily to patient safety improvement organizations that are designed solely for quality improvement and patient safety. It also seeks to create incentives for voluntary reporting systems that are non-punitive and promote learning. A "near" companion bill introduced in the U.S. House of Representatives (H.R. 4889) also states that if an organization believes it qualifies as a patient safety organization, under S. 2590, it can self-qualify to the Agency for Healthcare Research and Quality (AHRQ).

Risk Management Tips:

■ Peer review and quality improvement evidentiary protections vary from state to state and are further interpreted by state courts. It is imperative to seek initial and ongoing competent legal review of your organization's procedure for maintaining the confidentiality of FMEA documents.

■ Have the team chartered by the process improvement (PI) committee and the work performed under the auspices of the quality committee or, if applicable, under direction of legal counsel.

■ Evidentiary protections provided under state law should never be assumed. For example, it is possible that through the conduct of an organization or individual, that a court would consider an evidentiary privilege "waived" by a defendant, thus allowing peer review analysis such as a FMEA to come into evidence in a malpractice trial.

■ Consider limiting distribution of work product to avoid inadvertently waiving privilege. One way to limit distribution of FMEA work product is to bifurcate analytical work product (limited distribution) from written recommendations and implementation plans that receive wider internal distribution.

■ Until such protections can be assured at either the state or national level, providing a "disclaimer" or "intent statement" on a FMEA is recommended. Again, consult your organization's counsel.

■ Cite every page of a FMEA work product as "confidential" and with a statement of the intended privilege, whether it is a peer review privilege, quality improvement privilege, or attorney-client privilege. Consult legal counsel to select the appropriate citation.

As more proscriptive and refined approaches to understanding how errors occur in the healthcare environment are identified, risk managers appreciate that the FMEA process has the potential to provide a useful framework to enhance patient safety. Proactive risk assessment promotes decisions being made based upon the collection and analysis of data in the quest to proactively reduce potential harm to patients. Adopting a new approach can take time and will require patience, yet applying failure mode analysis can yield numerous opportunities for improving patient safety

SHARPENING THE TOOL: HOW TO OPTIMIZE FMEA

In getting started...

1. Seek support from senior leadership.
2. Seek out a trained facilitator or get training in facilitation. A good facilitator is important to open communication.
3. Help team members figure out what they will gain from the experience, involve them in developing a schedule, and give them ownership.
4. Look for best practices already identified for the process being assessed.

Index

AACN. *See* American Association of
    Colleges of Nursing (AACN)
Accreditation. *See also* Nursing
  evaluation process, external, 4
  quality potential level, continuous
    quality improvement (CQI), 5
  standards, 4
    patient safety processes, 150
  as voluntary process, 4
Accreditation Council for Graduate
    Medical Education (ACGME),
    88–89
Accredited health care organizations
  adverse events, reasons for, 83
  care specialization and silos, 91
  fatigue in workplace
    and medical errors, 89
    overtime, nurses, 89
    resident training, 88–89
    sleep deprivation, 89
    work shift, 89–90
  health care, reliability in
    aviation, 85
    CRM training, 86

high-reliability organizations
    (HROs), characteristics of, 86
  tight coupling, 85
high-reliability organizations
    (HROs)
  diagnostic errors, 87
  multilevel regression analysis, 87–88
  testing process errors, 87
injury underreporting, 88
nursing staffing issues
  floating practices, 93–94
  job dissatisfaction, 95
  legislation, 94
  models, 94
  Registered Nurse Safe Staffing
    Act of 2010, 94
  work environment, 93
reliability concepts
  preventable harm, 83–84
  Six Sigma, 84–85
  three-tiered strategy, 84
workplace
  communication, 91–92
  safety, 90–91

Nondisclosure of medical
mistakes, 203
*Normal Accidents: Living with High-
Risk Technologies*, 26, 85
Novice to Expert model, 207–208
NPSA. *See* National Patient Safety
Agency (NPSA)
NPSGs. *See* National Patient Safety
Goals (NPSGs)
NQF. *See* National Quality
Forum (NQF)
Nurse(s)
American Nurses Association
(ANA), 198
employee centeredness, 235,
247–248
executive, 80, 151
level, 241
front line of care, ethics on, 198
hierarchy importance, in change
efforts, 196–198
information-processing styles,
196–197
licensed practical nurse, 197
medical errors/bad behavior,
198–201
professional experience, AHRQ
on, 225–226
role issues, 199
scheduling (temporal factors),
AHRQ on, 226
staffing, 78–79, 224–225
Nursing
with accreditation efforts,
240–242
caring, 243
courage, 243
culture of safety, development of,
245–246
ethics, 243
executive level of, 241
functional nursing, 102–103
individual level, design at,
246–247

models, 244
of care, 173–174
modular nursing, 103–104
organizational structures, 243–244
patient centered/employee
centered, 247–248
patient-focused care, 104–105
and patient safety, cultural
competencies, 107–108
primary nursing, 104
process, five steps of, 223
salary, 80
staff, issues of, 93–95
system level, at design, 242–243
team, 103
team development
executive level, 245
microsystem level, 244, 245
values, 243
*Nursing Staff in Hospitals and Nursing
Homes: Is It Adequate?*, 28
Nursing workforce, 293

Occupational Safety and Health
Administration (OSHA),
90–91, 262
Occurrence (O), probability, 276
Office of Inspector General (OIG), 39
Office of the National Coordinator
for Health Care Information
Technology (ONC), 33
OHA. *See* Ontario Hospital
Association (OHA)
OIG. *See* Office of Inspector
General (OIG)
One-person model, 203
Online tools for patient safety, 14–15
Ontario Hospital Association
(OHA), 57
Open systems, 113, 115
Oppressed group issues, 199
Order read-back, 293
Organ donation, 296